CW00832185

WORKING WITH
STUTTERING

Dedication

For our families

WORKING WITH
STUTTERING

A PERSONAL CONSTRUCT
THERAPY APPROACH

ROSEMARIE HAYHOW MSc, MCST
CELIA LEVY BA, MCST

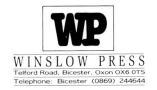

WINSLOW PRESS
Telford Road, Bicester, Oxon OX6 0TS
Telephone: Bicester (0869) 244644

First published in 1989 by
Winslow Press, Telford Road, Bicester, Oxon OX6 0TS

Copyright © R Hayhow & C Levy, 1989

All rights reserved. No part of this publication
may be reproduced, stored in a retrieval system,
or transmitted in any form or by any means,
electronic, mechanical, photocopying, recording or
otherwise, without the prior permission of the
Copyright owners.

Phototypeset by Gecko Limited, Bicester, Oxon

02–353/Printed in Great Britain by Hobbs the Printers,
Southampton

British Library Cataloguing in Publication Data
Hayhow, Rosemary
    Working with stuttering: a personal construct
    therapy approach.
    1. Man. Stuttering. Therapy
    I. Title   II. Levy, Celia
    616.85′5406

    ISBN 0–86388–068–1

CONTENTS

Rosemarie Hayhow MSc, MCST

Rosemarie Hayhow qualified as a speech therapist in 1969. In 1971 she joined a team of therapists at the City Lit in London, a centre specialising in the treatment of adults who stutter. She worked on intensive and evening courses and was involved in two research projects which evaluated, with the aid of personal construct procedures, the effectiveness of therapy. From 1977 to 1979 she was therapist in charge and also lectured on stuttering at the Central School of Speech and Drama, where she worked until 1986. Since the late seventies she has worked with disfluent children of all ages and has become increasingly interested in family therapy. She has completed courses in Personal Construct Psychology and Counselling and in Family Therapy. Currently she lectures in Cardiff and runs a clinic for children who stutter and their families.

Celia Levy BA, MCST

Celia Levy graduated as a speech and hearing therapist in 1971. She first became interested in stuttering therapy as a student and pursued this interest after qualifying. She joined the staff at the City Lit. in 1977 and later became head of the speech therapy department. She began studying Personal Construct Psychology (PCP) in 1981 and completed an advanced course in 1984. She has been involved in teaching stuttering therapy and PCP to both students and qualified therapists. In 1986 she organised a conference and subsequently edited a book reflecting British speech therapists' work in stuttering therapy*. In 1987 she became Senior Lecturer. Stuttering therapy is her main interest in speech therapy and she is currently researching how stuttering affects women.

*Levy, C (Ed) *Stuttering Therapies: Practical Approaches*, Croom Helm, 1987.

_____ EDITOR'S NOTE _____

For the sake of clarity alone, in this text we have used 'he' to refer to the client and 'she' to refer to the clinician, except in specific examples.

FOREWORD

Of the many books on stuttering produced each year often we can say that one is of interest. Occasionally we can rejoice that another has something new and significant to offer us. Only rarely are we invited to join in such a thoughtful and personal journey through the labyrinth of this area of human experience, as in *Working with Stuttering*.

The authors make no pretence that their journey has been an easy one or that it is now over. As clients will continue to experiment and grow, so will they and they invite us to make our own personal journeys, to make our own sense of what they have understood so far. The need for a comprehensive theory led them, as it has others, to Kelly's personal construct psychology. Through this complex but clearly articulated approach to the understanding of ourselves and others they are able to address many crucial issues in a coherent way: working with people rather than disorders; establishing the balance of responsibility between client and therapist; examining the aims of therapy and the implications of change.

As they take us step by step through every aspect of working with stuttering they make no sharp division between the 'psychological' and the 'behavioural'. The choice of fluency technique for a particular client is as much governed by their understanding of the client's view as is the choice of other experiments for change. The child's early experience of stuttering is regarded as part of their construing of themselves as a whole. Effective therapy is seen as having far more to do with a broader optimal functioning than simply a decrease in the number of syllables stuttered.

There is much practical as well as theoretical material here and ideas are presented in such a way as to be meaningful to experienced clinician and newly-qualified therapist alike. All can learn from the authors' reflexivity and the invitation to explore our own processes is implicit throughout the book, with a chapter devoted to self-experiment at the end. The authors are concerned to share not only their understanding of stuttering but the very real enrichment that personal construct theory has brought to their understanding of themselves and their roles as therapists.

The authors make it abundantly clear that this approach has wide implications for speech therapy, going far beyond the area of stuttering alone. Therapists have been slow to enlarge their horizons in their use of personal construct theory and, although this is a book about stuttering, its potential value in encouraging change in our approach to working with people as a whole is outstanding.

Peggy Dalton

PREFACE

Why we wrote this book

We first met in the spring of 1977, and since that time have worked together and collaborated in various ways. Recently we were reflecting on our experience as therapists and realised that between us we had worked with about 4000 people who stutter. We were aware that we had a wealth of experience that was informing our current approach to therapy and that the time had come to formalise our thinking in the shape of a book. Our motivation for writing this book was twofold: first, to clarify our theoretical assumptions about stuttering and therapy, and second, to share our experience in as accessible a way as possible with other therapists.

Because of the particular nature of our work, we have been fortunate in being able to focus on dealing only with stuttering. Further, because of our role as lecturers to students and post-graduate therapists, we have had easy access to journals and books. Living in London has afforded us the opportunity to meet other colleagues and to further our studies in areas of particular interest. We realise that other therapists are not always so fortunate. Therefore our aim in writing this book is to share the knowledge acquired through reading, clinical experience, association with colleagues and further study in a single, comprehensive approach to stuttering therapy. We ask therapists to recognise that this book represents experience acquired to date, and that we hope to continue to develop in both skills and understanding.

In what way is this book different from other books?

In our view one of the unusual features of this book is that the development of both therapist and client is considered important. Through personal experience we have found that reflecting upon ourselves both as therapists and as people has enabled us to grow. This book is not prescriptive: it will not tell you what to do and when to do it, but rather you will be invited to consider linking your understanding of clients to your choice of therapeutic intervention. All techniques and activities have a strong theoretical underpinning derived from personal construct theory (**Kelly**, 1955)[*]. This leaves us with a book that is neither purely a textbook nor a treatment programme.

How to use this book

In order to gain maximum benefit from this book, we recommend that before proceeding with therapy, therapists read the chapters in sequence. We

---

[*] Any future reference to Kelly that is undated will refer to **Kelly**, 1955.

recognise that some therapists work only with children or adults, and therefore may be less interested in certain parts of the book. Notwithstanding, we recommend that therapists read it all: most of the ideas are relevant and adaptable to clients of all ages. We advise therapists most strongly to work through and test out for themselves the ideas discussed in the book before using them with clients. Activities are designed to facilitate experiential learning on the part of clients. Therefore choice of activities for therapy needs to be based upon as complete an understanding as possible of clients and how they may change.

Therapists may find it helpful to use the book for group discussions. Activities can then be tried, evaluated and extended in such a learning/ support group. Reading the book may present a new way of looking at therapy with people who stutter. Working through the final chapter with colleagues will bring much of the book to life and facilitate experiental learning by therapists.

Outline of contents

In the first chapter, readers will find our points of departure: the assumptions underlying our approach to therapy. We hope that therapists will evaluate these critically and not accept them as statements of truth. In our estimation, this may engage therapists in a creative process of scrutinising their own implicit assumptions, and hence they will be in a good position to formulate their own theoretical stance.

Chapter two contains techniques for exploring clients' understanding of their problems. Many of these techniques are relevant to all people, not just those who stutter, and therefore we recommend that therapists practise using these ideas on themselves, friends and colleagues before using them with clients.

The process of change is described in *chapter three*. This focuses upon those aspects of personal construct theory that we have found particularly helpful in understanding and directing change in our clients. The contents may be new and possibly difficult for some therapists and one reading may not be sufficient. As these readers progress through the book, some of their difficulties may be clarified retrospectively. We hope that readers will not be disheartened at the apparent complexity of unfamiliar ideas. As we ourselves have learned about personal construct theory, each rereading has brought with it new insights and increased possibilities of application. The theory has become less daunting and more exciting with greater familiarity.

In *chapter four*, we focus upon understanding children and their families. Ways of gaining an appreciation of family strengths and problems are described. In this chapter the child is considered within the context of the family and not as a separate client. In *chapter five*, therapeutic interventions are described that are based upon the information accrued through the exploratory techniques of the previous chapter. Direct work with the child is also considered. These chapters are most relevant to working with children and their families; however adults also have experience of family life, and many of the ideas have application to their current family groups.

We move on to working with adults in *chapter six*, which describes how to formulate a transitive diagnosis leading on to planning for therapy. *Chapter seven* gives an account of current therapy techniques, but also includes a way of using Kelly's experimental approach when helping clients to modify their speech. Ideas for selecting an approach and therapy regime are included in this chapter.

Chapter eight gives a theoretical account of group therapy which is relevant to any therapy group. However the examples which illustrate the group process are drawn solely from stuttering groups. The second half of this chapter contains group activities which are ordered according to their usefulness at each particular stage of therapy.

The continuing process of change is discussed in *chapter nine*. Both the problems that might arise and ways of dealing with them are discussed. In more traditional texts this chapter would have been entitled 'maintenance', but because the personal construct theory view of people is that they are continually involved in a process of change, we found that term restricting.

Chapter ten is for you, the therapist. In some ways this chapter is perhaps the most important one, since it is through experiencing the personal relevance of a theory that a person is able to apply it with ease and conviction to helping others. The chapter aims not only to instruct, but to provide therapists with the opportunity to indulge in and enjoy the process of self-exploration and change.

The appendix before the bibliography contains a glossary of terms used in the book.

In conclusion, the principles of therapy contained in this book are relevant to all clients, not just those who stutter. We invite therapists to give us feedback about the value of the book to themselves and their clients.

Rosemarie Hayhow
Celia Levy

January 1989

CHAPTER 1
POINTS OF DEPARTURE

CHAPTER 1
POINTS OF DEPARTURE

The theory and therapy presented in this book is based primarily upon *The Psychology of Personal Constructs*, by **George Kelly**, Norton Press, New York, 1955. However Kelly did not elaborate his theory in relation to particular groups of clients, nor did he say a great deal about the development of construct systems. Because his focus was more upon the adult than the child, the family group was also under-represented in his theoretical discussions. This has meant that we have looked elsewhere in order to elaborate personal construct theory in relation both to children and adults who stutter. Our sources are various and include the writings of speech, family, group and psychotherapists, psychologists, our own clinical experience and all those other generous people who have taught us on courses, through conversation and by inviting us to observe their work.

These sources have provided us with the foundations for our work. In this chapter we discuss the ways they have influenced our thinking on certain key issues in stuttering therapy. The following chapters elaborate our perspectives upon stuttering, people and therapy.

The nature of stuttering

(a) Cause and development

The view that stuttering is caused by a multiplicity of factors is hard to dispute, given our present knowledge. These factors may be language based, environmentally induced or inherited and it is the interaction of these factors with the child and the family that will largely determine how communication develops. We have come to believe more and more that the ways in which the family and significant others *construe (see Appendix)* stuttering are influential in its development or failure to develop. Changes in parental attitudes and behaviour will often result in changes in the child's speaking. As stuttering becomes more central to the person's view of self so it becomes more significant when making predictions about self in relation to others. As stuttering clouds the person's social *predictions (see Appendix)*, so it needs to be viewed increasingly as a psychological as well as a mechanical problem.

(b) The variability of stuttering

We find that assessing severity of stuttering on the basis of observed behaviour gives an incomplete picture of the problem. **Sheehan** (1975) suggests that the three factors which constitute the problem of stuttering are: 'speech behaviour, speech anxiety, and perception of self' (p103). Personal construct theory leads us to seek dimensions or constructs along which stuttering may vary. Therefore we would like to propose that therapists use the following diagnostic constructs for identifying how stuttering affects people at the start of therapy and the avenues of movement potentially open to them.

stutters infrequently	stutters frequently
stutters mildly	stutters severely
silent blocks	stutters more openly
interiorised stuttering	exteriorised stuttering
disclosing stuttering is a relief	disclosing stuttering is catastrophic
lack of appropriate pausing	pauses appropriately
normal sounding fluency	rapid, disrhythmic fluency
negative attitude to self	positive attitude to self
negative attitude to stuttering	neutral attitude to stuttering
high avoidance	low avoidance
preoccupied by stuttering	not preoccupied
coping	depressed
socially isolated	satisfactory relationships

How clients rate themselves on these dimensions contributes as much to our understanding as our own ratings do.

(c) Solutions maintain the problem

The idea that a problem might be maintained by a person's attempts to solve it, is not new to speech therapists. The diagnosogenic theory of **Johnson et al.** (1959) saw the parents' attempted solutions as being responsible for the child's normal disfluencies developing into stuttering. Much of the work traditionally done with parents is based upon this theory and aims to stop them using their attempted solutions. Parents are advised against asking the child to stop, slow down and so on and it is assumed that they can respond positively to this advice. Similarly it is accepted that stuttering is likely to become more severe once the child starts to *try harder* to speak fluently (**Williams**, 1971). Stuttering is not the only problem that might be maintained by attempted solutions. Many of the problems that are encountered by family therapists can be viewed in this way. The recognition of a need to stop the cycle of problem → solution → problem led **Watzlawick et al.** (1967) to formulate a theory and practice that they termed Brief Therapy. Brief therapy attempts to change the ways in which people deal with their problems, rather than the problem behaviours themselves. Therapy which does not succeed in altering the ways that people deal with their problems may serve to maintain them. When progress is poor, instead of blaming the client, we could consider our role in maintaining the problem.

We are committed to finding ways of intervening more briefly and more effectively. This commitment leads us to question some of the assumptions upon which stuttering therapy is based.

(d) It is hard to change the things that we fear

Fear is considered to be a central component of stuttering. **Williams** (1979) describes four specific fears linked to stuttering: first, fear of being found out; second, fear of the never-ending block; third, fear of one stutter precipitating an avalanche of stuttering and fourth, fear of behavioural disintegration. The common factor linking these fears is uncertainty. In personal construct theory terms, when we cannot make sense of events we experience anxiety.

People who stutter may never have confronted the fears that they experience so often when speaking or, as **Sheehan** (1975) suggests, they develop a fear of the fear. The reality of what actually happens when they stutter is not checked against what they secretly dread happening. They feel anxious at the thought that they might suffer rejection, humiliation or a complete loss of face in front of their friends, colleagues and so on. The fact that they have friends and jobs does not reduce the anxiety experienced prior to stuttering. Sometimes we fail to generalise from the good things that happen to us: it is as if such events are isolated from the rest of our lives. For example, a woman who has spent ten or fifteen years at home bringing up children will feel unconfident if she believes that the skills she has developed are irrelevant to life outside the home. If, on the other hand, she believes that her skills of listening, organising, refraining from hasty judgements, entertaining children, supporting other mothers and all the rest are valuable and relevant to a variety of jobs she will approach a return to paid work in a very different way. In much the same way the person who stutters and who is able to benefit from positive experiences may well find that he speaks more fluently as he progresses in his work, enjoys satisfying relationships or perhaps excels in amateur dramatics. Not only is he more able to admit new elements to the realms of different constructs but he is also able to build bridges between the different clusters of constructs within his system.

There is another important issue that many clients raise. Some refer to it as a sort of optimism: each time they speak they hope that perhaps this time they will not stutter, even though they fear that they will. Many clients fail to use speech techniques when they anticipate stuttering, preferring to gamble on chance fluency. Since their optimism has been invalidated time and time again we need to seek an explanation as to why people persist with this gamble. It is possible that the acknowledgement of stuttering forces them to place themselves on the negative end of all those constructs that are implied by the *stuttering–fluent* construct, for example, construing themselves as *out of control, inferior, a loser* and so on. Seeing themselves so negatively is so unbearable that most develop ways of returning to a more comfortable position as quickly as possible. One way would be to reassure themselves that they are not really like other people who stutter (**Fransella**, 1968). Another would be to blame others so that the listener is seen as responsible for the stuttering, or perhaps they resolve to try harder with the speech technique, because if they followed instructions better they would not stutter. This removes the issue from core structures to more subordinate constructs about the mechanics of speech.

(e) Over-sensitivity

The majority of people who seek treatment for their stuttering feel badly about the way that they talk. Stuttering causes them to experience very negative emotions that can interfere with their pleasure in life. These negative emotions may seem out of proportion to the severity of the stuttering: the client has become hypersensitive to speech disruption. The therapeutic implications of over-sensitivity have been elaborated by **Van Riper** (1973) and **Sheehan** (1975) whose therapy approaches include work on desensitisation. We subscribe to their view that over-sensitivity is fundamental to the development and maintenance of stuttering and that work on desensitisation is essential, although it can be profoundly threatening. Desensitisation plays an important role in the 'stutter more fluently' therapies (**Gregory**, 1979) and can also be valuable in preparing the client for a 'speak more fluently' approach. The over-sensitivity to disfluency cannot be separated from the fear that we discussed in the previous section and this means that work on reducing anxiety must be included along with the toughening up work that Van Riper describes.

Therapy and change

(a) Theory vs eclecticism

It is interesting that working with people who stutter has made many therapists aware of the importance of having a theoretical framework upon which to base their work. This may be due in part to the complexity of the problem and the fact that it spans all age groups. It has not been possible for therapists to simplify the problem so that they can feel satisfied with a purely mechanistic approach. Also the ways individual clients respond to the same therapy can be so varied that any poorly conceived theories of stuttering will soon prove inadequate. It is perhaps the obvious impact that stuttering has upon a person's life that has made therapists look for a psychological theory to aid their understanding of the person who stutters.

We believe that a theoretical framework should help the therapist understand people in general and themselves and people who stutter in particular, and also provide a model for change. The theory must also help us to understand why and how speech therapy methods work, so that we are not forced into a position of eclecticism. Many theories that have been used in the past have precisely this shortcoming and so the therapist is forced to abandon her previous convictions or to try to distort the evidence so that she can continue with her current practices. Once a comprehensive theory has been found then the advantages are apparent: success and failure can be understood within the framework and what was previously inexplicable or put down to client shortcomings can now be understood. For example, within other models failure to generalise fluency outside the clinic may be attributed to lack of motivation or laziness. Using personal construct theory we may hypothesise that the client is unable to make predictions in difficult situations unless he behaves as he always has, that is, he stutters. So he will continue to stutter until he is able to begin to construe the situation and the construction processes of the people he encounters.

Knowing what to make of different therapy outcomes is one of the problems that face the eclectic therapist. Therapists, like their clients, need to be able to make predictions about therapy on the minute to minute level as well as in the long term. When therapy is based upon some theoretical framework both client and therapist can make sense of individual sessions in relation to the long-term therapy aims. Without this structure, therapy may be reduced to a random series of games and activities. We have both experienced offering this type of therapy and although it often was enjoyable and even seemed to be beneficial to some, we were plagued by feelings of inadequacy. We were dissatisfied with our role as facilitators of social skills and frustrated by our inability to understand our clients as people.

(b) First order and second order change

The idea of these two different orders of change was developed by **Watzlawick et al.** (1974). First order change focuses on altering the problem behaviours and not on changing attitudes. For example, the teaching of speech techniques represents solutions of the first order. Second order change, however, involves both the client and the therapist in reframing the problem so that a new set of alternatives becomes available. For example, if a child's stuttering is seen as an attempt to deflect parental disagreement by providing them with a common focus of concern the possible solutions include family therapy, marriage guidance or helping the child to cope with conflict. Teaching speech techniques would not solve the problem when viewed in this way. **Fransella** (1970) invited us to move from first order to second order solutions when she proposed that stuttering was not a symptom but a way of life.

Many therapists construe anxiety in physical terms and offer relaxation training as a solution. If we view anxiety psychologically instead of physically the solution will be of a different nature. When anxiety is seen as the inability to make useful predictions therapy will be directed to elaborating the client's view of self in relation to others.

(c) Where does change come from?

If we were able to provide a simple answer to this question there would probably be little need for this book. The answer is made more complicated when we ask what is to be changed. Are we seeking first order or second order changes? Do we want people to change the way they talk or the way they think or both? We agree with **Fransella** (1972) when she maintains that change is brought about both by what we think and by what we do and that it is artificial to separate the two. Fluency is pointless if stuttering is feared with an intensity that makes life miserable. Conversely thinking of stuttering as something that you do is of little help if you continue to experience it as a powerful spasm over which you have no control.

We also need to consider how we change people's minds. Is it through argument, education, the provision of new information or does it happen as a result of seeing things in a new way? In the following chapters these questions will be addressed and so we will satisfy ourselves with a rather general answer for the time being. We subscribe to the view expressed by **Procter and Walker** (1987) that changing and developing are fundamental human processes that can at times get blocked by repetitive cycles of construing and behaviour. If the cycle can be broken then the resourcefulness of the individuals will reappear. Kelly's view of people is optimistic: we seek to elaborate our construct systems so that our predictive abilities are expanding along with the increasing range of events that we choose to encounter.

Although we feel confident in the resourcefulness of most of the people with whom we work, unfortunately many have serious reservations about their capacity for change. Years of stuttering and failed therapy have served to prove the intractability of the problem and their own helplessness. Even when they are successful in other spheres of their lives they may be incapable of feeling optimistic about speaking.

(d) The client–therapist relationship

Kelly likened the client–therapist relationship to that of a research student and tutor. The student knows her subject in depth and the tutor has experience in research and its problems. Together they can explore difficulties and find solutions within a context of mutual respect. In the context of therapy it may take time for a relationship of equality to develop, since clients may not initially share our view of a partnership. They may be looking for someone who will relieve them of the burden of stuttering by taking responsibility for therapy. Alternatively, they may view stuttering as a sort of illness and therefore view the therapist as similar to a doctor in that a cure will be forthcoming. It is important that our clients' expectations are discovered and taken into account. Similarly, we must understand the implications for ourselves of an equal relationship with our clients since it may increase our vulnerability and open us up to unwelcome invalidation.

The different models adopted by professionals working with parents have been considered by **Cunningham and Davis** (1985, p10). In the expert model 'the parental role is only considered in so far as it is necessary to carry out instructions given by professionals in relation to their objectives'. The transplant model uses the parents as a resource. The professional retains the control over decision making while teaching the parents some of their skills. The value of the parents is recognised and the child is more likely to be viewed in the context of the family. The consumer model is more akin to the type of relationship that we favour. 'The parent is seen as having the right to decide and select what they believe is appropriate for their consumption' (p13).

Not all therapists will aim for the same sort of relationship with their clients; however the implications of the relationship that is favoured should be thought about. If there is inconsistency between the model that we use and our expectations of our clients then resentment and dissatisfaction seem inevitable.

(e) Not everyone is a stuttering therapist

We make this obvious statement because we believe that therapists can be put off working with people who stutter because of the nature of stuttering and a lack of support from colleagues. It can be threatening to work with people who are the same age or just a little older than ourselves and who are capable of asking difficult questions. When newly qualified this is especially true and many therapists seem to avoid treating people who stutter because of previous lack of support and uncertainty about what they should be doing. Some people are referred for intensive treatment, not because it is right for them but because their therapists lack confidence and expertise.

There are therapists who recognise that the majority of their clients have needs that extend beyond the mechanical or physical and into the psychological. Experience gained while taking a holistic approach towards other client groups should help when working with someone who stutters. Supervision and discussion groups can do much to support therapists even when the members work in different fields.

(f) The timing of therapy is critical

People are able to make better use of certain types of therapy at different times in their lives. Adults often refer themselves for therapy at times of crisis and sometimes it is wise to ask them to wait for therapy while they sort out these other issues. For example, we would not usually recommend starting intensive therapy with someone who is in the process of a distressing divorce settlement, although we might start individual weekly therapy. A short course of daily therapy might be indicated for someone whose work commitments have suddenly changed to include far more speaking.

Issues that need to be considered when arranging a course of therapy include ensuring that clients are able to make the necessary commitment of time and effort, that sorting out their speech and related problems is a priority, and that they have adequate support outside therapy to sustain them through the process of change.

(g) Life is not a hierarchy

There are times when, as therapists, we wish we could control events outside the therapy room. Real life is so much more varied and unpredictable than anything we can manufacture during therapy sessions. People engaged in weekly therapy may report events that they found traumatic and their inability to deal with these events threatens the progress made so far. Since we must accept that we have no control over people's lives we must help our clients to develop resources and more positive ways of evaluating themselves in real-life situations. The development of resourcefulness takes time and needs to start early on in therapy.

The person who stutters

(a) No two people are the same

The importance of the uniqueness of the individual is central to Kelly's theory. In his theoretical exposition he states that: 'Persons differ from each other in their constructions of events' (p55). In practice this means that we cannot assume that we know what life or events are like for another person. We need to understand the meanings that experiences have for the individual before we can say that we know them. The implications of this are that no two people who stutter will have had the same experiences and neither will they require exactly the same management. Similarly, no two therapists will be able to provide identical therapy and, furthermore, therapist and client will view the same therapeutic experience in different ways.

In case it sounds as though we are removing all structure, we must add that there will be similarities in the ways in which we and our clients view events because we may share the same cultural influences and in some cases may have led very similar lives. This does highlight the importance of spending more time learning about the meanings that events have for a person who comes from a different cultural or class background from our own.

We also know something of stuttering and how it influences people's lives. For the newly qualified therapist this knowledge is reassuring and she is likely to look for those things that validate the stereotype that she holds. As her experience with stuttering increases so we hope she will be able to use the stereotype in an increasingly propositional manner. In this way the differences between individual clients become the focus of attention and the need for the security of a stereotype diminishes. Once the therapist has learnt to tolerate the uncertainty that comes from viewing each new client as unique then she is free to enjoy the challenge of therapy.

(b) Stuttering therapy is for the person and not the stutter

We do not view stuttering therapy as being distinct from therapy with people who have other problems. All of the therapeutic models that we draw upon were designed with a range of human dilemmas in mind and therefore are theoretically as relevant to someone with a voice problem as to someone with a fluency problem. We argue that it is the sum total of the individual that governs the suitability of an approach and not just one aspect of their behaviour.

However, consideration of the person as well as the problem increases the load upon the therapist and so support and supervision become priorities. The therapist who uses personal construct therapy with conviction will have a commitment to increased understanding of self as well as others. In the long term this can compensate for the extra risks and hard work.

(c) Once a stutterer always a stutterer?

We believe that our interventions with young children and their families will usually lead to the development of normal fluency. In addition, we hope that parents will feel that they know how to handle any further episodes of disfluency and will know when and where to go for help, should they require it. We believe that some children are predisposed to stuttering and that this predisposition weakens gradually through maturation. For example, a child with delayed language development and several relatives who stutter may have both an environmental and physical predisposition which may continue to exert some influence throughout childhood. There are other children who experience alternating periods of fluency and disfluency and we have no way of predicting when the disfluent episodes will stop. Therefore therapy must assume that the stuttering will reappear and parents should be prepared for this. When a recurrence of stuttering fulfils predictions and parents feel confident that they know how to respond then it is less likely that the vicious circle of anxiety, guilt and stuttering will be resumed. What is encouraging is that often there is no return to stuttering and the parents feel more confident in responding to the various other problems that beset them in the early years of parenting.

Once stuttering has begun to influence a person's behaviour and the behaviour of others towards them, then therapy must take issues other than just fluency into account. Change becomes a more meaningful objective of therapy and it is sought in the client's ways of thinking as well as in behaviour. The *stuttering–fluency* construct will, it is hoped, become less central to their construing of others and alternative constructs opened up, such as *good communicator–poor communicator*. Freer communication is another important aim, so that people are more often able to say what they want to say when they want to say it. The ability to develop satisfying interpersonal relationships may also become a goal. We must add that we respect our clients' need for fluency and we are not trying to fob them off with some second-rate goals. What we argue for is a realistic appraisal of the likely effects of therapy and for an understanding that fluency is not the answer to all problems. The adoption of this wider view of stuttering has led clients along a slower but more permanent path of change.

Finally, over the years we have seen a return to stuttering in many of those clients who experienced long periods of fluency after intensive therapy. For some, a short course of therapy was enough to re-establish their fluency, but for others a different approach to the problem was needed because their fear of stuttering had never really abated even though they had experienced hundreds of hours of fluent speaking. It is not just being fluent that makes for long-term change but the ability to use the experience of fluency to change construing of self and others. This underlines yet again the importance of understanding that experience does not necessarily change a person's construing. In addition, the people who occupy important places in our clients' lives may also need to change their construing of them and their speaking, otherwise they may inadvertently invalidate new constructions.

(d) Therapy for life?

Although stuttering is a complex problem that seems extremely resistant to change we do not, as a rule, recommend regular, long-term therapy. Experience and research (**Helps and Dalton**, 1979) has led us to believe in the importance of maintaining contact after intensive work, but that the nature, content and frequency of sessions may change with time. Goals will vary with different stages in therapy and these goals need to be negotiated and clarified if short bouts of therapy are to be used. We argue in favour of very long-term contact, that is, at least five years for adult clients, but that during this time there should be long periods with very little contact.

Work with children is usually very much quicker but we would still recommend maintaining some contact for at least two years after the last episode of stuttering. A child who is maintaining fluency by the use of speech techniques may be at risk of stuttering again. If speaking situations are still construed in terms of the mechanics of speaking, then the change back to stuttering is possible. Therefore contact should be maintained for at least two years after the child is able to speak with normal fluency most of the time.

It is useful to apply these follow-up criteria when evaluating published results of therapy although unfortunately the quality of fluency after treatment is often not reported. It is particularly important when evaluating the effects of speech techniques used with children, since the aim is normal, fluent speech and this should be achieved in most cases. It is hoped that, over the next few years, there will be more developments in therapy that will help us to reduce treatment time while increasing our clients' successes, since many of the things that we are doing with our clients currently may serve to maintain, rather than diminish, their problem with communication.

Conclusion

We see our 'points of departure' as issues for debate. We invite therapists to discover their own assumptions, perhaps by criticising ours or by discussion with colleagues and clients. We acknowledge that you may find, as we did, that the process of formulating your assumptions may need to be preceded by writing a book!

CHAPTER 2
EXPLORATORY TECHNIQUES

CHAPTER 2
EXPLORATORY TECHNIQUES

Introduction

In this chapter the emphasis is on the techniques described by Kelly and developed by people working with clients who have a variety of problems. The word *exploratory* is used rather than *assessment* in order to convey a sense of the process of shared discovery, as opposed to fact finding. All of the procedures that we describe are most useful when carefully selected to suit the client and when the responses are understood within the framework of personal construct psychology. We argue that initial exploration should always be designed for the client. The procedures that follow will help the therapist understand something of the client's basic beliefs and the personal significance that events have for them. This understanding will help therapists select and apply an appropriate approach. Whatever we do with our clients we are more likely to be effective if we take account of the person as well as the stuttering.

The orientation that the therapist has towards clients and their problems will influence the sorts of questions that are asked, and hence the information obtained. The following general principles will help the reader understand a Kellian orientation.

Understanding meanings

We are more interested in the client's perceptions of experiences than in what actually happened. Any event will be construed differently by the different people involved, and we do not see ourselves as judges, deciding upon what is ultimately true. There are times when written questionnaires are helpful in obtaining background information, especially when the client stutters severely. However we have found that during face to face interviewing of clients it is better to rely on an outline of areas to be covered while following a hypotheses-making and -testing approach. In this way, the focus remains upon individual clients and the particular ways in which stuttering has affected them.

In addition, when meanings, rather than facts, are the focus of the interview clients may feel that they are being understood and not merely interrogated. When both client and therapist combine their resources to unravel the mystery of stuttering, they begin to develop a relationship of mutual trust and co-operation. If only facts are sought, the client may be alienated or may feel as though the therapist has a responsibility to provide a cure, which is a logical expectation when the therapist opts for the role of 'expert'.

(a) Aim for sufficient information

When interviewing adult clients it is particularly important to develop the skill of gaining the maximum amount of relevant information with the minimal amount of talking, since many clients with more severe problems will not be able to communicate very quickly. We cannot justify asking questions that do not lead to a greater understanding. Too much information can cloud rather than clarify the important issues.

(b) A credulous approach

When adopting a credulous stance we accept what our client tells us and we attempt to anticipate and predict, using some of their constructions. In a sense it is an exercise in imagination: we think and act **as if** our client's constructions were true and follow logically from each other. We may do this automatically when we attempt to comfort young children who have hurt themselves. If we are at all sensitive to their needs we do not force our constructions upon them, but rather try to see things from their point of view. Hence an acknowledgement of the hurt, offering physical comfort and some appropriate 'making better' tends to lead to a quicker resolution than a sharp 'stop crying, it's only a scratch'.

A client who stutters may keep referring to *success* as opposed to *failure*, so when they describe a situation we can make predictions using this particular construct. For example, the client may be dreading a social event that will necessitate meeting new people. When we know that each new person will be judged as fluent, and by implication as *successful*, then we can see that the client's anxiety arises from having to construe self as a *failure*, this being the inevitable consequence of stuttering. We can then make predictions about how we would feel and behave if we were in the client's situation.

A credulous approach involves more than acceptance: it is also a means of trying to use another's constructions to see what will happen. It is important to remember that we ask our clients to do the same: we offer them our professional and some personal constructions of events and actions and then ask them to behave 'as if' they were true.

(c) The therapeutic relationship

Neither the therapist nor the client is able to solve the problems alone. The client comes for therapy because previous solutions have failed; however this does not mean that there is automatically a commitment to the therapy on offer. Working towards a shared commitment may be the first step in therapy. The way that clients construe therapy and the therapist will depend upon past experiences and also their understanding of the problems: the same is true for the therapist. An acknowledgement of these preconceptions and clear statements of aims can help in the development of a mutually respectful relationship. It is important that we do not just pay lip-service to equal relationships: we must monitor all those subtle indicators of superiority: for example, keeping the client waiting, allowing phone calls to interrupt the session, asking lots of factual questions, giving advice, and so on.

It can be difficult to avoid the 'expert' role with clients who ask for our opinion or advice. We may find ourselves dishing out remedies before we have realised what is happening. Some clients are extremely skilful at handing over responsibility and we must be watchful if we are to avoid the trap of taking on too much of the responsibility for change. Similarly, it is easy to mistake collusion for credulous listening. It is not helpful to validate those constructions that are causing problems and so gentle questioning is often better than agreement. For example, a client may believe that an irritable boss causes the stuttering at work. Rather than agree that irritable people make us uneasy we can question the client to find other ways of construing the boss.

(d) Questions are an important tool

In the section on construct elicitation we shall look in detail at questioning as an exploratory technique. As a general principle it is best to avoid *why* questions since the answer is often 'I don't know' or 'if I knew I wouldn't be here'. It is interesting to monitor yourself and see when you ask or feel tempted to ask 'why' questions. You may find that they arise when you are confused and feeling threatened by your inability to resolve a problem, or perhaps when you want to force a client to agree with your own version of the problem. Asking 'why' of a client may emphasise their confusion. *What* and *how* questions encourage the client to focus upon specific behaviours and qualities rather than on the more abstract aspects of the problem. Kelly suggests that if we want to know what is wrong, ask the person, but cautions us to remember that 'A pat answer is the enemy to a fresh question' and 'A pat question is the enemy to a fresh answer'. This quotation very simply underlines the importance of thinking up questions appropriate to our individual clients.

(e) Assessment may lead to reconstruction

Ravenette (in press) asserts that 'Any intervention to assess is at the same time an opportunity to promote change. The first interview, and it may be the only one, should therefore always be seen as an occasion for potential change'. Exploration does not attempt to fix the person in time in the way that a photograph does, but is more like 'pausing' a video recording for careful analysis of the picture, while recognising that as soon as you release your finger it will continue to run on.

The aim of initial investigation is not just for the therapist to find answers, but for all participants to gain some additional understandings and to appreciate some new alternatives.

(f) Discovering similarities and differences

This means that we are always interested in what the client says and in what his answer denies. For example, if a client defines the problem as organic this may preclude taking account of psychological factors. We may understand something of the client's construct system as we learn how experiences are grouped in terms of similarities and differences. Two apparently different situations might be seen to have something in common when the parents tell us that the child always stutters in both.

(g) Allow sufficient time

Sometimes the process of exploration may free the client's thinking so that he is able to construe events or people in a looser manner than usual. This may be useful for promoting change, but can also lead to anxiety since making predictions may become more difficult. Hence it is important to tighten construing at the end of a session and this might be done by suggesting that the client sums up what has been learned. Similarly time must be allowed for regaining composure after the discussion of painful material. The responsibility for pacing the session lies with the therapist and she must defer the discussion of difficult material if there is insufficient time. This can be done respectfully so that the client is reassured that the content is not being rejected. The therapist can say something like, 'This is obviously an important issue for you and it would be a mistake to try to squeeze it into the end of the session. Perhaps you could make some notes for next time.' It is interesting that often clients will go away and think about the issue in the light of the previous session and on the next meeting wish to discuss their own resolutions.

(h) Attempted solutions

We have already discussed the relevance of this notion to stuttering, but have not considered the sorts of questions that can be asked to explore the attempted solutions that the client uses to tackle the problem. **Procter** (1985b) suggests questions to ask during family interviews that are relevant when the problem is stuttering:

- How have you been trying to solve the problem?
- When the problem occurs what do you do in order to try and stop it? prevent it?
- How well did that work?
- What else have you tried?
- What have other people suggested?
- Does your mother (husband, son, sister) know about this?
- What advice does she give you?
- When she says that what do you reply?
- What does your father do when your mother tries to help?
- Then how does your mother respond to that?

Someone who has difficulty speaking at work could be asked similar sorts of questions about their working environment. In fact the questions can be easily modified so that they are appropriate to a variety of different contexts.

(i) The language of the interview

It is often easier to begin to understand a person's construction of events if we use their words. The words that the client chooses to use will have a special personal meaning for them and if we change them we may well be changing the meaning. When we begin to establish a common language we also communicate our respect for the client's views and our willingness to see them as different from other people with the same problem.

Aims of initial exploration

Personal construct systems are complex and influenced by events and experiences. They are more a form of perpetual motion than a fixed structure. Therefore we cannot aim to know another person's constructs nor to have a definitive map of how they are organised and used. What we can do is learn enough about the constructions that the client places upon relevant events and people to be able to predict the channels along which change is most likely to occur and the manner in which this can be achieved. We must also understand the risks of change for our client so that we do not sabotage our therapeutic attempts by forcing too much change too quickly. Since we can never fully know someone, and especially not a client, then the aims must all be preceded by the words 'begin to'. This also serves to emphasise the importance of process and the need to modify therapy in the light of new material. Therefore the aims are *to begin to*:

1 Learn about the *content* of the client's personal construct system. This can be done by exploration of constructs or of constructions of experiences. **Ravenette** (in press) favours the latter with school-age children and asserts that:

> Just as problems in physics and chemistry may be resolved without necessarily isolating molecules and atoms, so may human problems be resolved without necessarily isolating a client's constructs, which are the units behind his constructions. Thus it is frequently more appropriate to look for the client's constructions and let his constructs look after themselves.

2 Understand how the client construes, not in terms of content but in terms of *process*: in other words the style of construing and the emotions experienced.

3 Appreciate the *structure* of the client's system so that we can differentiate between core (the essential 'I') and peripheral constructs. The way in which constructs cluster together and the bridges between these clusters can help us understand the implications of changes in behaviour or construing.

4 When we have some understanding of content, process and structure then we can begin to *formulate hypotheses about the nature of the client's problem*. This leads to the formulation of appropriate steps to be taken to facilitate change.

Diagnosis

We use this word to refer to the planning stage of therapy and not to the attempt to '. . . cram a whole live struggling client into a nosological category' (**Kelly**, 1955, p775). There are many ways in which the same set of facts can be construed and so one set of facts does not lead to one particular diagnosis. The word 'stutterer' tells us very little about a person and is a diagnosis that the average person in the street could make. It holds no implications for management. **Kelly** (1955, p779) identified six steps in diagnosis which he stated in colloquial fashion as follows:

1 Exactly what is peculiar about this client, when does he show it and where does it get him?

2 What does the client think about all this and what does he think he is trying to do?

3 What is the psychological view of the client's personal constructs?

4 In addition to the client himself, what is there to work with in the case?

5 Where does the client go next?

6 How is the client going to get well?

The procedures described in the following sections can be used to work through these diagnostic steps. It is not possible to identify procedures to deal with each step in turn, since many procedures help with more than one step. A repertory grid, for example, will help with steps two and three as well as giving some indications for five and six. There are other issues to be addressed during the diagnostic stage and these will be raised in relation to the different procedures.

(a) Elicitation of personal constructs

Constructs are bipolar discriminations that we make in order to anticipate events and hence they structure our experiences. Construing is not the same as verbal formulation. Although we are able to find verbal labels that approximate to some constructs, there are many more that we will never verbalise. Constructs may be *pre-verbal*, in the sense that they were developed before language skills were sufficiently developed to express them; or they may be *non-verbal*, being to do with physiological processes. Even when we have mature verbal skills we still construe through our senses and constructs to do with smell, taste, touch and so on may be implied by other more verbally accessible constructs. This means that when we elicit constructs we must be aware that we obtain only a small sample, and that we need to know how these constructs are used if we are to begin to get some real sense of the person's construct system.

Constructs vary in their importance and in the extent to which they are used. The constructs that help an individual to define himself are the *core* or *superordinate* constructs and these are relatively few in number and difficult to change. Each system has many more subordinate constructs and changes in these do not necessarily imply change for the essential self. When eliciting constructs we hope to sample some of the core constructs so that we know something of the person's central values, fears and conflicts and how these relate to their problem. This raises the question of how we recognise core constructs. There is one very simple answer: we can ask, 'How important is this construct for how you think about yourself and others?' (**Leitner**, 1985 p300). People usually know when they have verbalised an important construct: they sense a ring of truth.

It is important to appreciate that it can be relatively easy to reach these essential constructions. For example we can ask a person whether they would rather live on a planet where they were totally ignored, or on a planet where they were always treated with hostility and aggression (**Rowe**, 1983). Asking someone to choose between these options sounds rather like a party game; however, when therapists try to find the answer for themselves they will quickly appreciate the seriousness of the question. Similarly, the procedures that we describe may take the interviewee very rapidly from a *subordinate* construct to the *reason for life*. Many people are not in the habit of sharing these highly personal beliefs with others and we must be careful not to abuse these powerful procedures. We may wish to glimpse a person's core construing so that we can better understand the meanings that experiences have for him and also so that we can avoid suggesting changes that will be too threatening. However, when we do this we are taking a risk. As we begin to understand our client's core construing so we open ourselves to the threat, anxiety, hostility, guilt and fear that are associated with the central self. **Leitner** (1985, p302) used the word 'terror' when discussing the risks of really understanding another person: '. . . any investigation into the core of the person may be terrifying for both the subject and the experimenter'.

It is much easier for the therapist and client to interact at a subordinate level although both may know that the problem is just being skirted around. This was brought home very clearly by one client who failed to make any progress with modifying his stutter. One day, perhaps more by chance than design, the client was able to verbalise some of his desperate hatred of himself and his stutter. The acceptance of this man's profound depression and of his need to explore the darker areas of his construing led to the eventual reconstruction of himself as someone who was worthy of love and respect. Only then was he able to begin to use the fluency techniques with which he had been struggling.

Finally, we advise therapists to try all of these procedures before they are used with clients. Suggestions for activities for therapists are listed in the final chapter; however, the procedures are described here. We hope that therapists working together will find the procedures interesting and useful and thereby gain sufficient confidence and competence to begin to use them with clients. A respect for the other person's view of the world will ensure that the understandings gained while working together will not in any way be misused. The apparent ease of elicitation of constructs should not be taken as an indication of their superficiality.

In our experience, these techniques provide powerful ways of exploring another's view of the world. Most clients who are committed to the notion of increasing their understanding of self and others find the process interesting and exciting. They will feel threatened at times, but when this is acknowledged and understood within the context of the person's construct system then it may mark the beginning of some alternative constructions. The emphasis is upon exploring meanings and not upon the therapist placing her constructions upon the client's experiences.

(i) Eliciting constructs from elements

An element is the term given to the things, events or people that we construe. The terms 'construct' and 'element' have been introduced as two different ideas; however, this is not accurate. **Fransella and Bannister** (1977, p11) remind us that: 'There is no such thing as an element that is *only* an element or a construct that is *nothing but* a construct. Thus, *father–not father* can be used as a dimension along which other people are placed, as being *father–like* or *not father–like*. But 'father' can also be an element construed in terms of, say, the dimension *strong in character–weak in character.'*

Constructs can be elicited from any elements but it is usual to select ones that represent the area under exploration. Kelly suggests twenty-four role titles from which to select elements when personal relationships are the area of interest.

1 A teacher you liked (or the teacher of a subject you liked).

2 A teacher you disliked (or the teacher of a subject you disliked).

3 Your wife, husband or present girl/boy friend.

4 An employer, supervisor, or officer under whom you worked and whom you found it hard to get along with (or someone under whom you worked in a situation you did not like).

5 An employer, supervisor, or officer under whom you worked and whom you liked (or someone under whom you worked in a situation you liked).

6 Your mother (or the person who has played the part of a mother in your life).

7 Your father (or the person who has played the part of a father in your life).

8 Your brother nearest your age (or the person who has been most like a brother).

9 Your sister nearest your age (or the person who has been most like a sister).

10 A person with whom you have worked who was easy to get along with.

11 A person with whom you have worked who was hard to understand.

12 A neighbour with whom you get along well.

13 A neighbour whom you find hard to understand.

14 A boy you got along well with when you were in secondary school (or when you were sixteen).

15 A girl you got along well with when you were in secondary school (or when you were sixteen).

16 A boy you did not like when you were in secondary school (or when you were sixteen).

17 A girl you did not like when you were in secondary school (or when you were sixteen).

18 A person of your own sex whom you would enjoy having as a companion on a trip.

19 A person of your own sex whom you would dislike having as a companion on a trip.

20 A person with whom you have been closely associated recently who appears to dislike you.

21 The person whom you would most like to be of help to (or whom you feel most sorry for).

22 The most intelligent person whom you know personally.

23 The most successful person whom you know personally.

24 The most interesting person whom you know personally.

When eliciting constructs from a client who stutters, some of the above role titles can be used and it may also be useful to use some or all of the following:

1 As I am now;

2 As I'd like to be;

3 As I am when speaking fluently;

4 As I am when stuttering;

5 As I used to be;

6 As I think I will be after therapy.

The traditional method for eliciting constructs is through the presentation of triads of elements. Three are selected and the client is asked to think of an important way in which two are alike and thereby different from the third. This response is recorded and the client is then asked how the third person, thing or event is different, thus supplying the contrast pole. After presenting a couple of triads, clients will often be able to state both ends of the construct as they consider the different people. This can be facilitated by having the elements on separate cards so that they can be moved about on the table. For example, the client may move 'mother' and 'as I am' close together and separate from 'brother' while saying that mother and self are *considerate* and brother is *selfish*.

Some clients, especially children, may find it easier to specify the differences or similarities between any two elements. Occasionally the idea of 'similar to and different from' causes problems for the client, in which case a single element can be presented. The client is then asked to think of a word that best describes the single element and then to think of the opposite.

There is no set number of constructs that can be elicited from elements: the therapist must decide how many triads are appropriate and when or if to move on to some other method for eliciting further constructs.

(ii) Elicitation of constructs by laddering

Constructs are organised hierarchically, that is, some are superordinate and subsume the more subordinate constructs. For example, the constructs *kind—unkind* and *liked—disliked* may both be subsumed by (subordinate to) the construct *needs people—isolated*. If we are to understand the meanings that events have for a person, it is important that we sample superordinate as well as subordinate constructs. A procedure for doing this was first described by **Hinkle** (1965) and termed 'laddering'. The steps are as follows: select a construct that has been elicited by means of a triad or other procedure described in this chapter. As an example we will consider the construct *stutters—speaks fluently*. Throughout the laddering procedure it is important that the client understands that it is his personal reasons that are required and not some accepted logic. The subsequent steps will now be presented in dialogue form:

Therapist: Which of these would you prefer to be, a person who *stutters* or a person who *speaks fluently?*

Client: I'd prefer to *speak fluently.*

This now becomes the preferred pole.

Therapist: Why would **you** prefer to be the sort of person who *speaks fluently?*

Client: Because then I can say what I want to.

Therapist: Whereas if you *stutter?*

Client: Then I can only say certain things.

Therapist: What do you see as the advantage for **you** in being able to say what you want to?

Client: I can be a more effective speaker.

Therapist: Whereas if you can only say certain things?

Client: Then I'm less effective.

Therapist: Why would **you** rather be an effective speaker?

Client: People will listen to me.

Therapist: Whereas if you are a less effective speaker?

Client: You get little feedback.

Therapist: So what are the advantages for **you** of being listened to?

Client: I can share with others and make friends.

Therapist: Whereas if you get little feedback?

Client: I will become isolated.

Therapist: Why is it important for **you** to share with others and make friends?

Client: Well, without relationships there's no point really.

This example helps us to understand why the client feels so depressed by his stuttering. It is obvious when the top of the hierarchy has been reached since the final answer is a sort of philosophical statement, one of the person's reasons for living. There is no required number of steps to be taken to reach the top of a hierarchy although eliciting more than six constructs becomes tedious and may indicate that the person is not giving their own reasons but rather trying either to please or to challenge the therapist.

(iii) Pyramid procedure

This procedure is, in a sense, the opposite to laddering: it takes us down the hierarchy, becoming more concrete. It was developed by **Landfield** (1971) not for assessment, but rather with psychotherapy in mind. The elaboration of constructs that occurs can be used to increase understanding, to identify problematic constructs and to provide the starting-point for change. In their discussion of the pyramid procedure, **Landfield and Epting** (1987) suggest that the client is asked

> . . . to think of an acquaintance with whom he feels most comfortable and whose company he most enjoys. The clinician does not ask for the name of the acquaintance, but he may ask if it is a male or a female. The client is then asked to give a brief (several words) description of his acquaintance, focusing on the person's *one* most important quality or characteristic. (p65)

The therapist may request that the client thinks of a person who has some other effect upon him, for example, an admired person or someone who makes the client feel inferior. Once the client has decided upon an important characteristic, it is no longer necessary to consider the person just described. The client is then asked for the opposite to the quality just elicited and this establishes the construct at the top of the pyramid. The therapist now works from each of these poles. Starting with the first, the client is asked what kind of person has this characteristic. Once this similarity is established the client is asked to state the kind of person who is most different. This establishes the first construct at the second level of the pyramid. Next the client is asked, in the same way, about the other pole of the first construct so that there are two constructs at the second level. The same procedure can be carried out with the second level leading to four constructs at the third level.

Landfield and Epting suggest that one or more of the following questions be asked about the different responses. If we take *trusting* as an example, we might ask: 'How would you know if a person was trusting or alternatively not trusting; when would a person be trusting or not trusting; what might a

Figure 2.1 An example of a 'pyramid'

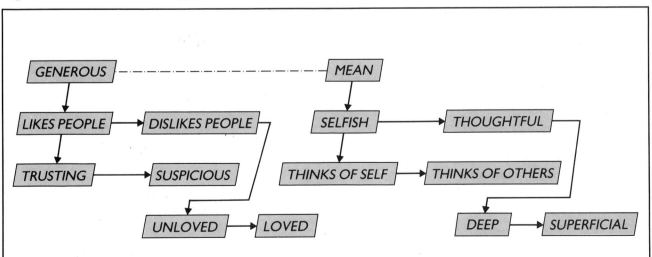

trusting person say, think or feel?' Questions of this sort help the therapist understand more about the behaviours that are governed by the constructs under discussion. They might also serve to reduce anxiety in a client who is finding the focus on constructs too abstract or too challenging to their present ways of construing people.

It is possible that the client will be surprised to learn that some constructs keep recurring during laddering or pyramiding. This is potentially threatening since the client may begin to doubt the usefulness of the recurring constructs. When this happens the person may feel at a loss, their ability to predict is reduced and they may sense impending chaos. If we are sensitive to this and discourage the client from contemplating rapid change, then the threat can be reduced and some of the aims of therapy clarified. Relating constructs to specific behaviours is a tightening procedure that makes life more predictable again.

(iv) Elicitation of constructs during structured conversation

Whenever we discuss clients' problems, attitudes towards work, friendships and so on, or specific significant events, we are learning something of the constructions that are placed upon experiences and by implication learning about important constructs. However if our aim is to elicit constructs then we must be sure that we have the right verbal labels for both poles. It is possible that we are mistaken when we believe we understand our clients and so we should routinely check our understanding with them. When we are listening to a client and aiming to understand more of the meanings that events have, then we are listening for themes, notions that recur and points where difficulty or frustration are verbalised. Because of the bipolarity of constructs we are interested in what the client says and also in what the response denies. As we begin to build up an idea of what is important to the client so we test this by asking appropriate questions. Some of the examples of questions given below have been suggested by **Procter** (1985b).

- 'In what way are these two similar?' or 'In what way are the two of you different?' are the type of questions that help to establish differences and similarities and can be useful not only for the elicitation of personal constructs but also for exploring their significance.

- 'What do you do when you feel depressed (anxious, etc)?' helps the therapist to understand the impact that feelings have upon the person's life as well as to explore coping strategies. A question phrased in this way also implies acceptance by the therapist.

- 'How do you know that . . . devalues you because of your stutter?' may reveal great difficulty in making sense of other people's behaviour as well as the client's over-use of a *stuttering–fluency* construct.

- 'What is the opposite to . . .?' can be used in a variety of forms to obtain the implicit pole of a construct. To elaborate the rarely used end one can ask, for example, 'What would be different if you were fluent?', 'How would you recognise approval from a listener?'

- 'How will you know when you've improved?' and 'What must happen so that you can feel satisfied with the way you talk?' helps us to understand what clients will accept as validating and also how they view the problem. If clients see stuttering as a sort of illness then they may well look for a cure. If they see it as a physical problem then they may talk about practice and gaining control. Alternatively if they emphasise the psychological component of stuttering they may talk about changing attitudes and feelings. **Procter** (1985a, p333) discusses the prevalence of 'medical understandings of psychological problems' where the referred client is seen as *ill* in relation to the rest of the family who are *well*. There may also be a *good—bad* construct that leads to ideas of punishment, laziness or confusion: 'I try to lead a good life, so why has this stutter happened to me?' It is helpful to understand the superordinate constructs that govern the way the problem is viewed if therapist and client are to share therapy goals.

There are other types of questions that encourage the sort of discussion that helps the therapist understand the client's view. **Landfield and Epting** (1987, p87) suggest using the following as springboards for discussion:

■ **Magic wand:** If you could transform yourself what would you become? It is likely that the answer will indicate a dimension along which the client would like to move but finds that he cannot.

■ **Decisions:** The client is asked to talk about decisions that might have been made, ones he wishes he could make and some he is glad he did not make. The client is encouraged to focus upon the feelings as well as the thoughts that are associated with these decisions.

■ **Life span:** How have you changed over the last few years? Have you changed your feelings about things over the last few years?

■ **Same and different:** How are you the same as and different from other important people in your life?

Leitner (1985) found three topics of discussion that elicited core constructs. He stresses the importance of a good relationship between therapist and client because of the personal significance of the content that arises. This means that these topics are not usually suitable for a first meeting.

■ **God:** Constructions of God are of central importance to a religious person and so if we wish to understand them we must understand their construction of God. **Rowe** (1983) also stresses the importance of people's religious beliefs and the need to understand how they fit with the presenting problem.

■ **Significant** (life-turning) **events:** These are not necessarily the events that others would recognise as being significant. They may have to do with life, death, partings and unions or may be apparently trivial; for example, a chance remark or even a funny event that suddenly offered an alternative view.

■ **Mile-post dream:** Vivid, realistic dreams that the dreamer finds memorable and significant may well mark a change in the client's construct system.

These different starting-points for discussion should be selected according to the interests of the client as well as the aims of the session. It must be remembered that the material they produce is likely to be of greater personal significance than the client might anticipate. So not only must time be allowed for full discussion but also for a return to more subordinate construing before the client leaves the session. Helping the client to construe the themes that have arisen during the session serves to close the discussion. Focusing on events expected in the week ahead enables clients to leave with an anticipatory framework.

(b) Self characterisation

The self characterisation is a means of helping the therapist enter the personal world of the client. Analysis of the sketch may suggest possible ways of helping the client change their view of themselves and their problem. These possibilities emerge as clinical hypotheses, which can be tested by the client and therapist in the course of therapy.

In order to experience how our clients view their world, we need momentarily to suspend our own view of life and credulously absorb the writings of our client. This implies a non-evaluative approach, which pays equal attention to all the information offered, no matter how insignificant it may seem at first. We try and behave 'as if' everything the client has written is true and real in their own terms.

The instructions for the self characterisation have been carefully worded to reduce threat and anxiety.

> I want you to write a character sketch of Harry Brown, just as if he were the principal character in a play. Write it as it might be written by a friend who knew him very intimately and very sympathetically, perhaps better than anyone could ever really know him. Be sure to write it in the third person. For example, start out by saying 'Harry Brown is . . .'. (**Kelly**, 1955, p323)

A self characterisation is rarely analysed in the absence of other information about the client and their construction processes. It offers a very different perspective since the client is invited to take an overview of their life which contrasts sharply with the procedures already described, which encourage a focus on specific constructs. A self characterisation provides an opportunity to see how the client's constructs help the individual make sense of self. If clients produce lengthy sketches it may be helpful to ask them to summarise the main themes.

Some ways of analysing the self characterisation

- Look out for topic sentences, often at the beginning of paragraphs. Very often the first sentence is important. Somewhere in the final paragraph there is usually another important sentence.
- Try to identify the themes that run through the sketch.
- Try and understand the meaning of each sentence in the context of the whole sketch: that is, if the rest of the sketch were an explanation of this particular sentence, what does this statement mean?
- Look out for words or phrases that are repeated. These are likely to be important constructs which the client uses to differentiate self from others.
- Read each sentence shifting the emphasis on the words, so that you do not impose your own meaning on the writing.
- Try and restate each theme in your own words. This really helps you take on the role of the client.
- Make a note of the topics mentioned. This helps to see the areas in which the client characteristically identifies himself. Also note which areas are not mentioned.
- Assume that the whole sketch represents a true continuity. Apparent breaks can be seen as either an elaboration of the opposite pole, or the expansion of subjectively similar material.

It is important to bear in mind that writing a self characterisation is often very difficult and represents a very personal account of self. It is a document that needs to be treated with great respect and the utmost confidentiality. The points given above will make more sense when they can be discussed within a supervision or study group. We recommend that therapists write their own characterisation and analyse it before attempting one with a client.

When a client finds writing difficult the sketch can either be dictated to the therapist or spoken into a tape-recorder. There is no definite lower age limit; however it may not be a realistic task for children of less than about nine years of age. (See *chapter 4* and *chapter 6* for examples of self characterisations.)

(c) Elaborating the complaint

The ABC Model (**Tschudi**, 1977) helps to clarify the conflicts that may hinder change along a particular construct dimension. It is usual that once a problem has been identified the individual is able to discuss why they wish to change. However, there may be other, less desirable changes that are implicated and of which the person has little awareness. When these implicative dilemmas are explored the personal cost of change can be assessed. Sometimes it is realised that the cost is too great and that change is therefore no longer desirable. More often it becomes apparent that exploration of different ways of construing the problem and its possible solutions is required. It is hoped that it will then be possible to change without suffering the negative consequences.

Figure 2.2 A way of writing down the ABC Model

a1	Tactless	a2	Tactful
b1	Likely to hurt someone	b2	Able to show sensitivity
c2	Get a chance to say what you really mean	c1	Have to hide your true feelings

The procedure for exploring the advantages and disadvantages of a particular change is given below:

1. Define the problem that you wish to explore, for example, an embarrassing situation where you said something you wish you had not. Allow yourself to think freely for a few minutes. Write down all aspects of yourself that were at stake in that situation. It is important to keep to the context of this situation only. From your list pick one word or phrase that seems central to the cause of your embarrassment. In this case such a word might be *tactless*. We call this a1.

2. Find the opposite of this, which might be how you would have liked to behave. The word might be *tactful*. This becomes a2.

3. You now have construct A, which defines the axis along which you moved in the embarrassing situation.

4. List the disadvantages of a1. There may be only one, or quite a few. Once you have your list, pick the most important one, which we will call b1. In this case it might be *likely to hurt someone*. Now list the advantages of a2, again picking the most important one. This is likely to be the opposite of b1, in this instance, *able to show sensitivity*. This is construct B.

5 Now you can look for the reasons why it might be difficult to change. Consider the advantages of a1, which we call c2. Here the advantage of being *tactless* might be that you get a chance to *say what you really mean*.

6 Now consider the disadvantages of a2, which we call c1. In this example, the disadvantage of being *tactful* might be *having to hide your true feelings*.

This person will have to resolve the dilemma that exists between showing sensitivity and yet being able to say what she really means. Are there tactful ways of expressing real feelings? Perhaps learning to be assertive would enable this person to be more open without being hurtful.

(d) Repertory grid technique

This technique enables the client and therapist to see how a sample of constructs are used in relation to a particular group of elements. The particular elements chosen will be determined by the questions that the therapist wishes to explore and usually these will include some self elements and some from Kelly's list of role titles. The range of convenience of the constructs should include the selected elements and sample both subordinate and superordinate construing. The range of convenience of a construct comprises all those things that can be discriminated between, using the particular construct. The construct *fast—slow* can be applied to cars, animals and so on but makes less sense when applied to people unless they are a group of people whose speed is a crucial characteristic, like athletes or racing drivers. This means that the range of convenience is not a fixed phenomenon but rather dependent upon the particular elements and the area of enquiry. Some constructs have a wider range of convenience, for example, *good—bad*, whereas others have a much smaller range, for example, *makes me look thin—makes me look fat*, which can only be applied easily to certain clothes and funny mirrors. Constructs that do not include the selected elements within their range of convenience will distort the grid data.

Another factor to consider is the individual's use of a construct. An interesting example is provided in **Fransela and Bannister** (1977) when they describe a man who restricted his use of an *attractive–unattractive* construct to women. He was able to differentiate between women on the basis of attractiveness but he rated all men as unattractive. Therefore the inclusion of this construct in a grid would distort the picture of his system.

There is some controversy about the use of supplied constructs, that is, constructs that are thought to be appropriate to the client but not actually elicited from them. The use of supplied constructs might be justified when research requires that different people's grids are compared; however, we would not recommend the practice when exploring an individual's construct system.

The size of grid will depend upon the methods of analysis and the tenacity of the client. A popular size is somewhere between 14 by 14 and 18 by 18. When first using grids we suggest having one element more or less than constructs, which ensures that constructs and elements cannot be confused on the computer print out.

The method of grid completion will depend upon the client's age and abilities. Different ways of conceptualising the task have been developed for different age groups and for clients with a range of different communication problems. In general, the aim is for each element to be rated or ranked for each construct. Recommended rating scales vary from a minimum of 1–3 to a maximum of 1–9. When working with adult clients who understand the task, we have found either a 1–7 or 1–9 scale most useful. Clients are usually able to discover for themselves which scale they prefer. Once a client has conceptualised the grid task it may be possible to complete the grid in the form shown in *chapter six*, page 106.

Other clients, particularly children or those with comprehension difficulties, may need to have each element presented separately so that they have pages with all the constructs written and one element at the top. Each point in the rating scale may need to be labelled.

Figure 2.3   Presentation of a single element, a labelled rating scale and a sample of constructs

Best Friend							
	very	quite	a bit	neither	a bit	quite	very	
happy								sad
cold								warm
satisfied								angry
timid								brave

Grid technique is not a test and so does not require a rigid adherence to a particular form of administration. What is important, though, is that both therapist and client understand the task and the reasons for doing it. The most interesting and useful ways of eliciting constructs and completing grids can then be found. Some clients may wish to talk as they complete the grid and this allows the therapist to gain insight into the thinking behind the ratings that are used. Others may find this inhibiting and therefore prefer to work quietly on their own, only discussing those points that are either particularly difficult or interesting.

It is not appropriate to talk about the validity of grid technique in the way that we discuss the validity of a questionnaire. Grid technique is not an assessment that claims to measure particular traits or characteristics, but rather it provides a way of looking at the relationships and patterns that exist between constructs and between elements. The value of this information is determined by the appropriateness of the constructs and the elements that are included and by the questions that are asked of the data. If constructs are elicited in a careless, hurried fashion or if the therapist takes responsibility for finalising the verbal labels the client may have difficulty in rating elements. This may become apparent when the pattern of rating reveals over-use of the middle rating point, suggesting that the constructs do not help the client to discriminate between the elements. However, when constructs have been elicited with care and elements chosen to fall within their range of convenience, we may learn much from the resulting grid data.

A grid does not provide a 'true' picture of a person's construct system. Firstly, it would not be possible to convert a whole system into one small grid, and secondly, people do not stay the same or always see things in the same way from one occasion to the next. However, if the procedure is meaningful, there should be consistency at a superordinate level. If the grid helps us to understand how the client's problem fits with their view of self and others and also gives some indication of how change might occur then it is a justifiable procedure. In addition, many clients find that the process of construct elicitation clarifies or elaborates issues around the problem. The grid then becomes a therapeutic procedure as much as an exploratory one.

Sometimes the tasks of construct elicitation or grid completion do not seem meaningful to the client. Ratings seem arbitrary and the client is obviously not engaged in the process. When this happens we should question our use of the procedures, their appropriateness to the client at the current time and the meaning that the difficulty could have for them. For example, someone who is construing in a loose manner may not be able to tolerate the tightening that grid completion enforces. Others may use the constructs in a random manner because insufficient care was taken to ensure that personal constructs, rather than adjectives and their opposites, were elicited. For example, when laddering constructs we must ensure that the client realises that it is the importance that things have for *them* that interests us, not some generally accepted logic. Whatever data we get from grid procedures we must keep asking what it *means* and not focus upon the apparent 'truth' of it.

There are different computer programs available for the analysis of grid data and they all have accompanying manuals that explain the statistical methods used and the resulting print-out. The Centre for Personal Construct Psychology has information on currently available grid programs and their address is given at the end of the chapter. Whichever program is used, the onus is upon the therapist to think of questions to ask of the data. Some of the questions that we have found useful are given below and we hope these are sufficient to stimulate the reader into thinking of more.

1 How many components are there for both constructs and elements? This gives us an indication of whether the person relies upon one cluster of constructs for making sense of other people. At the other extreme, there may be a lack of structure, so that knowing a few things about a person does not help the individual make useful anticipations.

2 Can you find a theme that the constructs of each component have in common? In this way we understand more about the client's core construing: these themes are of great personal importance.

3 How are the elements grouped? Is there a theme covering each cluster of elements? With clients who stutter, speaking and control or success are often important themes.

4 Are there a lot of significant correlations, or only a few? How do you explain this?

5 Has the data thrown any light on the way the person wishes to change? Compare elements such as 'me now' with 'as I'd like to be'.

6 Can you find any reasons why the person may find it difficult to change?

7 How does the person construe self in relation to others?

8 If you were taking this person on for therapy, where would it be easiest to help the person begin to change?

We recommend that therapists complete and analyse a grid before attempting one with a client. The process of construct elicitation and grid completion can then be appreciated and the difference between this and a 'test' should become very clear. When the data is one's own questions may spring to mind more easily than when struggling to make sense of a very different view of life.

Conclusion

The exploratory procedures outlined in this chapter all aim to increase our understandings of a person's view of the world. This means that they can all be practised on self and colleagues before being used with clients. Although many of the techniques seem simple this must not be taken to reflect their superficiality. Any information gained must be treated with the utmost confidence and respect. This means that we should not use these procedures for the sake of appearing competent but rather we must carefully select them to match the particular client and the questions that we have in mind. Familiarity with the techniques and the information that they elicit will enable therapists to select appropriately. As each session is evaluated we may find answers to some of our original questions. This process generates further questions which can be explored in future sessions. It is the questions to which we seek an answer that provide the framework for exploratory sessions.

These procedures are not designed to compare clients either with each other or with a 'normal' population. As we formulate hypotheses concerning the client and the problem so we can begin to select appropriate techniques. The therapist does not aim to be an objective observer of the client but rather a companion on a journey of discovery.

Further references

Beail, N, *Repertory Grid Technique and Personal Constructs: Applications in Clinical and Educational Settings*, Croom Helm, London, 1985.

Fransella, F and **Bannister, D,** *A Manual for Repertory Grid Technique*, Academic Press, London, 1977.

Landfield, AW and **Epting, F,** *Personal Construct Psychology: Clinical and Personality Assessment*, Human Sciences Press, New York, 1987.

The Centre for Personal Construct Psychology, 132 Warwick Way, London SW1V 4JD. Tel *01-834 8875*

The Centre has a collection of personal construct theory research projects, books and articles in their library. They are able to provide information on the software available for analysing different types of grids. In addition, they run courses on PCT.

THE PROCESS
OF CHANGE

Chapter 3
THE PROCESS
OF CHANGE

In this chapter we would like to explore the process of change with the focus on the person who comes for help. Although written in the context of a book on stuttering therapy, this chapter is about the broader issues of change and will, we hope, provide therapists with an understanding of how to facilitate change in all clients.

The need for a theory

In most training establishments speech therapy is taught disorder by disorder. Therefore student speech therapists may never develop a theory about people that enables them to make equal sense of all their clients, regardless of their speech problem. Further the theories they evolve to understand clients with different communication problems may be of little use when looking at their own behaviour. Turning to psychology may not help either, for there too the student will find that reductionism runs rife. Take a look at the headings in most psychology texts and you will find the person split into processes: memory, learning, perception, thinking and so on. Once qualified, therapists may cling to the techniques they were taught for each disorder to give their therapy structure, even if the ideas underlying them are incompatible with each other.

As therapists we need a theory which will enable us to make predictions about all people, whether they have problems or not. 'A theory may be considered as a way of binding together a multitude of facts so that one may comprehend them all at once' (**Kelly**, 1955, p18). Consider the advantages for the therapist who has a professional system of ideas that exist at a sufficiently high level of abstraction that, whether she is working with a dysphasic adult or a child who stutters, she can refer to this one comprehensive body of knowledge to plan a process of change for her clients. Contrast this with an eclectic approach which forces us to borrow ideas from here and there without necessarily having a deeper understanding of their theoretical assumptions.

Personal construct theory

Many stuttering therapists have been drawn to personal construct psychology (PCT) because of the work of **Fransella** (1972) with adults who stutter. However, an erroneous association between stuttering and PCT has crept into our thinking. We seem to believe mistakenly that PCT is a theory about stuttering that has no generality to the other work we do. PCT is first and foremost a theory about the individual, any individual, and it has broad relevance to ourselves, our clients, our friends and our families.

What is personal construct theory all about? **Kelly** (1955) based his theory on a philosophical idea which he called 'constructive alternativism'. To restate his philosophy, 'there is nothing in the world which is not subject to some form of reconstruction' (p937). The implication of this is that even though reality exists, there are many possible ways of construing it. Some of these are better than others in that 'they support more precise and more accurate predictions about more events' (p15). To date we do not have a universal theory that can account for all things. As a species we are engaged in the continual process of refining and evaluating our personal theories until they approximate to reality with greater efficiency. This philosophical position even allows for the eventual replacement of PCT if another theory is devised that leads to better predictions of events.

Kelly's view of the person is different from other psychologies. 'Psychoanalytic theories suggest that man is essentially a battlefield, he is a dark cellar in which a maiden aunt and a sex-crazed monkey are locked in mortal combat, the affair being refereed by a rather nervous bank clerk' (**Bannister**, 1966, p363). The learning theory perspective is that we are born as a blank slate with the capacity to learn and remember. Everything we do (that is, all behaviour) is viewed as a result of reinforcement or punishment contingent upon the responses we emit in relation to stimuli. In contrast, Kelly conceptualises the person as a scientist who generates hypotheses to predict events, tests these out and evaluates the results.

The basis of our predictions is the construct, which is a way in which some things are seen as being alike and yet different from others. When faced with a continuous stream of events we note that certain events repeat each other. When we have abstracted the particular property that makes an event similar in some way to a previous occurrence, we have the basis for a prediction. For example, by abstracting the properties of *light vs dark*, we are able to construe the difference between day and night, and to predict that one follows the other. If we are unable to find a way of making sense of events, we face chaos. Therefore construing is our way of structuring reality.

To this end we each evolve for ourselves a system of constructs which we organise in a very personal way. Some of our constructs are likely to be very concrete and therefore are useful for predicting everyday events and interpersonal interactions. These constructs tend to be subordinate to constructs that are pitched at a more abstract level. The superordinate constructs subsume the more subordinate ones and are useful for making sense of broader issues. For example, the construct *stuttered speech—fluent speech* is subordinate to the construct *poor communicator—good communicator*. Speech therapy techniques are often directed towards the more subordinate level, that is, the establishment of fluency. However, when we evaluate our therapy, it is likely that we will need to refer to more superordinate constructs to decide how successfully the person is using the technique. Subordinate constructs have fewer implications than their more superordinate counterparts. Because subordinate constructs tend to be good for predicting a more limited range of events, we are likely to require a greater number than of superordinate constructs.

It may be useful to imagine that a personal construct system resembles a pyramidal structure. At the bottom are the subordinate constructs, and proceeding upwards are the highly organised lines of reference to the more superordinate constructs. At various levels on the way up there may be horizontal linkages between subsystems of constructs. The more superordinate a construct is, the more resistant to change it is likely to be (**Hinkle**, 1965). Thus if a client uses the construct *stuttering—fluency* as the basis for almost all predictions about himself in relation to others, because of the huge investment in the meaning of this construct, it is likely to be very resistant to change. Another client, with ways of judging himself other than by giving pride of place to the *stuttering—fluency* construct, is likely to be able to change his speech more easily.

As indicated earlier, constructs form the basis of predictions. When we discover that our predictions are accurate, that is, that there is compatibility between the prediction and outcome, then the prediction has been validated. We have a construct that we are likely to be able to use again to anticipate similar events. If there is incompatibility between our prediction and the actual outcome, then our prediction has been invalidated. Perhaps we will have to revise our construct, or try again, but more of that later. Kelly believed that people are primarily concerned with the anticipation of events. We are not being driven by repressed forces; we are not being pulled by the carrot of reinforcement. 'Anticipation is both the push and pull of the psychology of personal constructs' (p49). The goal is control. But because the universe does not stay put, for it too is evolving, we may never create a system of constructs that will be good for all time. Therefore we engage in a constant process of testing the preciseness of fit of our constructs. We never stop construing and therefore we never stop changing.

Accounting for change

One of the most usual ways of accounting for change is in terms of change over time. **Salmon** (1985b) points out that developmental psychologists would have us believe that after birth we are engaged in a continuous process of change until we reach our twenties. By this stage they believe we have 'developed' and that through our adult years life seems to stand still psychologically. But their interest in us is reawakened when we reach 'old age'. Late human life is treated as the loss of everything gained in early life: in fact, the mirror image of early development. The psychology of ageing is becoming increasingly important as more and more people outlive their three score years and ten.

Kelly believes that life is most conveniently plotted against the continuum of time, resulting in a view of the person as changing from one moment to the next. Even construing can be considered to be a sequence of events. To Kelly, the person is a form of motion, ever reaching for the future, never standing still:

> ... life is a way of using the present to link the future with the past in some original fashion. (**Kelly**, 1980, p28)

If we accept Kelly's view of the person as being constantly engaged in the process of change, then accounting for development in terms of age, milestones, phases or stages of development seems less meaningful.

Change is far from passive, for construing is the active process of making sense of the situations in which we find ourselves, experience being that which is construed. As new information is taken on board, the person's construct system is revised. Therefore younger children differ from older ones both in the smaller number of constructs in their repertoire and also in the lesser degree of organisation in their sytems. This relative lack of organisation has the advantage of rendering the younger child's construct system more amenable to change (**Salmon**, 1970).

The permeability of the system, that is, the extent to which a construct is able to absorb new elements into its framework, is a further means of accounting for change. In early life, the child develops constructs which help her anticipate her parents. If these constructs are permeable, the child will find them useful when trying to make sense of other people she encounters. **Salmon** (1970) gives the example of the early construct, 'like my mother' which changes to 'motherly' as the child successively uses it to discriminate between adults in her world. As a construct admits new elements within its range it is likely to vary both in its structure and the verbal labels used to describe the discrimination being made.

Bannister and Agnew (1977) were interested in discovering how we develop a notion of ourselves as individuals. They studied children of five, seven and nine years and found that the older children were able to differentiate what they had said four months previously from what other children had said by using psychological inferences such as 'That child said he wanted to be a soldier and I could never kill anybody so I wouldn't have said that' (**Jackson and Bannister,** p68, 1985a). This contrasted sharply with the younger children who tried to remember what they had said and, if they could, were able to identify themselves. They concluded that 'our construing of ourselves is developed as a bipolar construct of 'self versus others' and that the whole construct elaborates in the same way, and as part of, the system whereby we construe the world at large' (**Bannister and Fransella,** 1986, p74).

In a fascinating study which compares children who are seen as 'problems' with 'good' children, **Jackson and Bannister** (1985a) found many differences in the construing processes of older and younger children, some of which are given below:

1 Older children used more psychological cause and effect statements than younger children.

2 Older children were more able to anticipate accurately how others would rate them than younger children.

3 As children get older, they are more able to predict how members of their peer group may behave.

4 The construct systems of older children were more complex and organised than those of younger children.

The children in this study were 9–10 years old in the younger group, and 12–13 years old in the older group.

Children judged as 'problems' by their teachers tended to have less well-developed construing of self and others than their 'good' counterparts. Further, they were considered to be harder to understand by their peers. The importance of these findings for us is that when we are referred children who are causing concern, part of our therapy may need to be directed to helping these children elaborate their construing of self versus others.

Because personal construct theory views life as a form of motion, using the term 'development' is somewhat misleading. 'It implies movement towards some end product, whereas there is no such concept within the psychology of personal constructs' (**Bannister and Fransella,** 1986, p85). Therefore we need to examine the process of change in a different way. The headings that follow may be unfamiliar landmarks for some readers. We invite you to stay credulous, reading what we have to say with the question ever-present in your mind, 'If this were true, how would it change what I already know?'

Behaviour is the experiment

Most psychological theories regard behaviour as the response to a stimulus, but not so in the pyschology of personal constructs. **Kelly** (1970) viewed behaviour as our principal instrument of inquiry.

35

Personal constructs form the basis of predictions which we make in order to control the course of events. Having made a prediction, we must test its predictive accuracy, and behaviour is the means to this end. Through our behaviour we commit ourselves to our inquiry about some matter, then we collect the evidence and can review how well our prediction worked: our cycle of experience is complete. This contrasts with a learning theory view of behaviour, which would have us behaving in ways we have behaved before because of the favourable consequences. Kelly sees [man's] behaviour as anticipatory and original. 'When he acts he poses a question, and what ensues gives the question its import, the act its potency, and his life its meaning' (**Kelly,** 1969, p36).

Take as an example a man who finds himself in a field where there is known to be quicksand. He has to get across the field. As he looks at the ground in front of him, he does not know if it will bear his weight. He chooses a likely patch, and tentatively puts his foot forward, not knowing until he takes the step what will happen. He moves forward gradually, each time testing the consequences of his predictions. Bit by bit he construes the replications of events: clumps of grass are more likely to support him than bare patches of sand. Meanwhile, unknown to him, a woman is watching him from a distance. She knows nothing of the quicksand and attributes his peculiar movements to superstition or craziness. She may even smile because it looks so funny. Unless she understands what experiment the man is conducting, what question he is asking each time he takes a step, she will not be able to make sense of his behaviour. Her first thoughts are that his behaviour is a consequence of his madness: she does not understand that it is a means to an end.

Let us apply these ideas to stuttering. Suppose a child stutters every time his parents argue. One way of looking at this behaviour would be to see the stuttering as a response to the tension he feels when his parents argue, (the stimulus). A Kellian therapist would ask herself what experiment the child is conducting by stuttering at these times. Looked at from the child's point of view, the results of stuttering might be very validating. Instead of arguing, the parents focus on the child and so stuttering could be seen to maintain the *status quo* in the home. He has engaged in an experiment which works according to his view of the situation. Stuttering is likely to persist because it stops his parents arguing with each other and unites them in their efforts to help him. The behaviour has meaning for the child when viewed in this way. We are not proposing that this is thought out and planned at a high level of awareness: it is more likely that the experiment was taking place at a non-verbal level.

As therapists, if we try to understand the nature of the experiment a person is conducting when they stutter, our therapy will be very different from that of therapists who view stuttering as a reaction to stress. Such therapists might teach relaxation, or work on the symptom itself. A Kellian therapist would try to help the person reconstrue. If the therapist hypothesised that a child was trying to stop his parents arguing, as in the example above, she might discuss with the child why people argue and try to elaborate his construing of arguing, with the hope of enabling the child to conduct a different experiment the next time his parents quarrel.

Perhaps the child sees arguing leading to the breakup of his home. He may hear his parents say things like, 'I don't know why I stay with you'. If indeed the marriage is on the point of breaking up, the therapist may refer the family for therapy. However, suppose the arguing has no dire implications for the family, except that it distresses the child; then the therapist would be free to help the child to view arguing in a different way. To be theoretical for a moment: when a person views a problem in a particular way, one set of alternatives might be apparent to him. In this instance the child sees arguing as the beginning of the end of his family life. His choice of tactics for dealing with this stems from his view of the situation: his parents are focused on each other, but if he can distract them, they will focus on him instead. His choices might be: being very naughty, stuttering, screaming or crying. If a person can be helped to view the problem differently, other alternatives are possible (**Procter and Walker,** 1987). In this example, the child might learn that it is possible to feel angry and argue without stopping loving that person. He could be invited to think of times when he feels angry with his brother/sister or parents, but still loves them. He could take comfort from the fact that his parents do not leave after they have quarrelled. This view opens up other alternatives: the child can ignore his parents, leave the room, ask them not to make so much noise and so on. Through the elaboration of his view of the situation, his original construction of the situation has been invalidated, and therefore stuttering is unlikely to persist. Alternatively, work with the parents could lead them to understand the implications of arguing from the child's point of view. They could try to find other ways of settling their differences.

In personal construct theory, behaviour is seen as an integral part of the cycle of experience. Action without thinking is not deemed possible, since our actions stem from our view of a situation. Thinking without action, although possible, would not lead us anywhere, since the only way we can evaluate the intellectual manipulation of our constructs is through a behavioural enterprise.

Levels of awareness

Kelly has chosen to reject the concept of 'the unconscious' along with terms like 'motivation', 'repression' and 'defence mechanisms'. In his opinion people are in the business of making sense of their lives: the search for understanding is the very stuff of life itself. However he acknowledges that we do not carry all of our past constructions in the forefront of our awareness: we are able to construe before we have language, sometimes we are unable to gain access to some of our personal constructs and sometimes we forget experiences. If this is not repression at work, how might we understand these processes within the psychology of personal constructs?

(a) Pre-verbal constructs

These are constructs which continue to be used although they have no consistent word symbol. Pre-verbal constructs originate in infancy and are usually to do with sustenance or dependency, both of which are crucial issues in a baby's life. As the child grows up, verbal labels often conceal pre-verbal construing. Therapists may encounter evidence of pre-verbal construing in clients who become very dependent during the process of therapy. The flood of words may disguise the presence of pre-verbal construing. For example, 'I've heard such good things about you. I'm sure you are going to help me. I just know this therapy will work'. It is likely that something about the therapist is evocative of a parental figure. Alternatively, needing help may remind them vividly of their early dependency relationships.

(b) Submergence

When one pole of a construct is less available than the other, we may hypothesise that it is submerged, Consider the client who says, 'Everyone rejects me'. Only by understanding the opposite can we fully appreciate the meaning of this construct. Various possibilities exist: perhaps the client is saying, 'No matter how hard I try to make people like me, everyone rejects me'. If this were so the clue would lie in the client's behaviour. In such a case, the client would be friendly, ingratiating and needy.

Suppose the client were saying, 'Everyone rejects me, but I reject no one'? In this instance, the client would be placing himself on the submerged pole of the construct, using the construct to differentiate between himself and others. If a construct has a submerged end, it is less available for testing. When this client was asked how he construed the people he found so rejecting, his response was circuitous: 'I want everyone to like me'. When challenged further, he replied that he had never considered how *he* felt about other people, only how they felt about him. As this pole is made more explicit, it may have threatening implications for the client, involving him in reconstruing himself in fundamental ways. He may find, for example, that he does not like the people who reject him, invalidating the assertion that he rejects no one.

(c) Suspension

In order for an event to be remembered, it must be slotted away along some or other construct dimension. Over time our personal construct systems change and we are likely to replace old constructs with new ones that better meet the demands of our present lives. If some of the elements subsumed by these constructs do not get absorbed into the new constructs they may drop out and disappear. These elements are said to be suspended, and will only be remembered when they can be admitted into the range of convenience of a new construct. For example, when buying toys for a five-year-old, we may find ourselves remembering the toys we had as children as we hurriedly search for constructs to enable us to choose an appropriate present.

Kelly is careful to emphasise that forgetting is not due to repression. Rather 'one remembers what is structured and forgets what is unstructured' (p473). The process of therapy, particularly if it is directed to exploration of the past, is likely to help clients to remember events that they had forgotten. If these have been painful, perhaps viewing them through the new constructs emerging in therapy will help the client to reconstrue them. For example, during desensitisation in block modification therapy, many old wounds are reopened by exploring feelings linked to stuttering. Bad reactions such as laughter or ridicule are likely to be remembered. When seen through adult eyes, clients can be helped to understand that a listener may have laughed through ignorance and insensitivity, and to let some of the hurt and anger go. Asking clients what they would like to have said to such people at the time can help them deal with the hurtful situation from the present.

(d) Levels of cognitive awareness

As mentioned earlier, it would be impossible for us to hold all of our experience in our minds at once. Kelly proposed a scalar type of construct to give us a way of viewing our construing. He called it the level of cognitive awareness. The diagnostic constructs of pre-verbal construing, submergence and suspension represent a low level of cognitive awareness. Constructs which are easy to verbalise, and whose alternatives are accessible, represent a higher level of cognitive awareness.

Take for example a client who is always fluent with certain people, but cannot readily say why. In looking at their similarities and differences, the client may discover that all these people are 'mother-like' figures. The prediction of fluency is based on construing at a low level of awareness. Contrast this with a client who can specify the phoneme, the syllable stress and the place in the sentence of words likely to evoke stuttering. We may assume that such construing is at a high level of awareness.

Individuality, commonality and sociality

The emphasis thus far has been on the uniqueness of the individual. Indeed, Kelly was at pains to stress the fact that our view of the world, and therefore our behaviour in relation to it, arises from our personal interpretation of events, Because we are each at the centre of our own stage, experiencing other people as external figures, we may differ from each other in our constructions of events. The implication of this is that no two people can have the same experience, no matter how closely associated they are. This is apparent in families, when children are exposed to the same circumstances and each responds differently.

However life would be somewhat chaotic if there were no common ground. Kelly accounts for commonality, where he hypothesises that if two people (or more) anticipate events in similar ways, their psychological processes will duplicate each other. Stating it the other way around, Kelly asserts 'that two persons' psychological processes will be as similar as their constructions of experience' (1955, p91). People are similar to the extent that they derive the same meaning from an experience.

In this way Kelly accounts for similarities in people's behaviour. For instance, Kelly postulated that cultural similarity derives from a similarity in what people perceive is expected of them. 'People belong to the same cultural group, not merely because they behave alike, nor because they expect the same things of others, but especially because they construe their experience in the same way' (**Kelly**, 1955, p91).

Neither the construct of individuality nor the construct of commonality completely accounts for the way we become ourselves. The ways in which we construe others, and the ways we construe their constructions of us, are the building blocks of our social roles, Our personalities are the result of continuous anticipatory effort. Our role in relation to others is based on the extent to which we are able to construe their construction processes.

Two people who meet for the first time are involved in a process of construing each other so that each may adjust themselves to the behaviour of the other. When a therapist and client meet, each tries to assess the construction processes of the other so that they may conform to the role that is expected of them. The source of validation or invalidation lies in the social sphere. A newly qualified therapist may be anxious to have the respect of her client, and will try to find out what impresses the client. It may be that she has to make profound statements about the nature of the diagnosis, or that she has to listen very carefully, or write extensive notes and so on. She can only find this out through trying to see things through her client's eyes. The client, on the other hand, may wish to reserve judgement until he has changed in some way. However, when he sees that the therapist is seeking validation, he may decide that there is a better chance that she will help him if he responds positively to her efforts.

Neither person would be behaving in this way, save for the presence of the other person. And here we come to Kelly's somewhat different understanding of the term 'role'. For him, a role is 'an ongoing pattern of behaviour that follows from a person's understanding of how the others who are associated with him in his task think' (p98). The role we play in relation to others derives from our personal anticipations of others. It is an active, changing process, which is not dependent on commonality between construction systems.

Playing a role in relation to a person need not be based on correct mutual understanding. Family life often throws up examples where individuals assume that they see things the same way, and show little understanding of each other as a consequence. For example, father and five-year-old son go to the cinema one evening. On the way out, they pass a bar in the foyer, and the child asks for a drink. The father refuses and the child promptly throws a tantrum. In the father's mind was the notion that the child had had enough treats for one day and, as it was late, they should be getting home. The child was seeing things differently: up to that point he was being treated as a grown-up, and the refusal of the drink was powerfully invalidating. Suddenly he was a child again; his experiment squashed.

The three areas of individuality, commonality and sociality have profound implications for change. Individuality gives us the responsibility and the awesome task of inventing and reinventing ourselves. For therapists, its importance cannot be overestimated. No two clients can be assumed to be 'the same', and each person who comes for help should sense that their individuality is both respected and taken into account in the planning of therapy.

Commonality has important implications as well. Therapists may reach greater understanding of a problem such as stuttering by looking at similarities and differences between clients. Further, an understanding of what is expected of the client by others, that is, the context in which he hopes to change, will influence the course of therapy. For example, a client who was an important businessman sought help. His stuttering was more interiorised, and because of the success of Sheehan's approach-avoidance therapy with similar clients, the therapist was inclined to recommend this approach to him. However, as she attended to what he wanted from therapy, and the fact that his colleagues at work were demanding fluency, it became apparent that open stuttering would only be possible if his colleagues could be involved in the therapy process. In the end, a fluency approach with work on desensitisation to stuttering was chosen as the best place to start.

An understanding of sociality is vital in stuttering therapy, where the stuttering can be seen to be part of the role a person plays in relation to his listener. Many clients are fluent with speech therapists, even if they do not know the first thing about them as people. In the same way, they may stutter with authority figures, members of the opposite sex or with any person they cannot construe adequately and therefore focus on speech production to give the interaction structure. If we are to help our clients to experiment with different roles, we need to understand how they construe others' constructions of them. In group therapy, clients can be helped to find alternative roles in relation to others if the therapist views the construct of sociality as anticipatory rather than as a product of past reinforcements. Role is not fixed, but an ever-changing way of testing our social predictions.

Choice

Our personal construct systems afford us both our freedom and our limitation. We are free to the extent that it is possible to construe events in a number of ways. However, because we evolve systems of constructs to anticipate most circumstances that we encounter, only a limited number of pathways or movements may seem possible to us.

When we are faced with the need to make a choice, Kelly predicts that we are likely to choose that alternative which seems to provide the best basis for anticipating events. The choice may extend or define our system, making it more comprehensive or more explicit and clear. In the final stages, our choice is confined to a particular construct, and we must choose between these two alternatives to precipitate ourselves into action.

For example, when going shopping for clothes, we may browse in shops for a long time, looking at different dresses. Finally we narrow down our choice to a few garments. We may have used several personal constructs, such as *suitable for the occasion—unsuitable* or *affordable—too expensive* to reach this stage. When we make the final choice and buy the dress, we home in on one pole of one construct, which then pushes us off the edge of speculation and into action, for instance: *this dress really suits me*. If the dress is very unusual, we may be in the process of extending our system, venturing into new territory. If the dress is like others we have, we may be clarifying and defining our taste.

It is worth noting that we do not necessarily make wise choices. If we have a fixed and inflexible view of the situation, the alternatives which suggest themselves to us may be limited. On the other hand, if we feel that anything is possible, it may be impossible to make a choice. Kelly describes the cycle of decision making or CPC cycle as follows:

- **Circumspection:** during this phase the person is able to consider various possibilities and explore their consequences without any commitment to action.

- **Pre-emption:** now the possibilities are narrowed to a single construct, which limits the choice to two alternatives.

- **Control:** the person chooses 'that alternative through which he anticipates the greater possibility for extension and definition of his system'. (p517)

In order to understand the choices a client has made, or might make, the therapist needs to know both the content and structure of the client's personal construct system. Directing clients to take a course of action is unlikely to help unless it has some meaning for them, that is, it extends or defines their systems. It is possible that relapse in stuttering therapy is attributable in part to the fact that the tasks we require our clients to perform are not construable by them and therefore do not lead to the better anticipation of events.

Summary

In both this and the previous chapter we have covered some of the important theoretical concepts underlying the process of change. These may be grouped under three main headings:

1 **Content of the personal construct system:** this includes the verbal labels of constructs. Procedures for eliciting constructs were described in *Chapter Two*.

2 **Structure of the personal construct system:** included here are concepts such as core and peripheral constructs, comprehensive and incidental constructs, subordinate and superordinate constructs, changes in structure over time.

3 **Process of construing:** the key words covering this area are behaviour is the experiment, anticipation, levels of awareness, individuality, commonality, sociality, choice and decision making.

When a person changes in any way, each of these three areas is implicated. Changes in the content of construing are likely to have come about through behavioural experiments and as new constructs or elements are incorporated into the system so the structure of the system will be affected.

There is a fourth factor which accounts for change which we will call **style of construing**. Again this has implications for all three areas described above, but is especially linked to the process of construing. The headings that follow all describe the ways in which we may use our personal constructs.

Tight and loose constructs

When we make predictions we may use our personal constructs in different ways. *'Tight constructs are those which lead to unvarying predictions'* (**Kelly,** 1955, p483; our emphasis). All the elements which lie within the range of convenience of the construct are consistently construed at one end of the construct or the other. An example common to many people who stutter is the way in which the construct *stutterer–fluent speaker* is used. Speakers tend to be consistently classified as exemplifying one pole or the other. Therapists may challenge a client's use of this construct by asking clients to think of instances when they stuttered but felt calm and relaxed, to all intents and purposes like a fluent speaker.

'Loose constructs are those which lead to varying predictions' (**Kelly,** p484; our emphasis). Sometimes an element is construed at one end of a construct, and sometimes at another. A construct such as *happy–sad* may lead to varying predictions, with people being construed sometimes at one pole, and at other times at the opposite pole.

Creativity stems from alternating between loosened and tightened constructions. At first we may have a hazy idea of the methods we might employ to solve a particular problem. We may need to think laterally and loosen relationships between constructs that were previously closely related. Suddenly, and in a flash, we arrive at the solution. We have tightened our construing and have a prediction that we can put to the test. It is hard to fathom where the idea came from — we may have been day-dreaming, taking a leisurely bath and not even thinking about the problem, when suddenly we realise we have cracked it.

In order to be creative we need both phases of loosened and tightened construction. If we used our constructs loosely all the time we could not be creative. We would live forever in a dream world and never set up hypotheses to test. Eventually we would lose touch with reality. Drugs may produce loosened construing, and some people may turn to drugs when they lose inspiration and cannot get away from their tightened ways of viewing the world. A person who consistently uses tight constructions may be very productive, but will not be creative. For example, librarians may classify thousands of books each week according to the strict rules of their system. Each day produces more of the same. 'Creativity arises out of preposterous thinking' (p529).

In therapy change is brought about by the creativity of both the therapist and the client. Each must be able to alternately loosen and tighten their construing. Careful control must be kept over this process. Too much loosening and the client may get lost in a dream world. Too much tightening and the client does little but define the problem with greater and greater clarity and yet does not change in relation to it.

Most people feel more comfortable with one style of construing than the other. Some clients have a great need for certainty, accurate predictions and control, factors which the therapist will need to take into account when planning a process of change. Other clients seem much more flexible and unconcerned with the outcomes of experiments. They may approach therapy as the intellectual manipulation of constructs, but never act on their new ways of seeing things. Such clients may benefit from some tightening before they can make use of therapy.

Therapists too may have a preference for generally looser or tighter constructions. A therapist who is happier with a looser style may find the need for certainty expressed by a 'tight' client profoundly irritating. No doubt the converse is equally probable. We believe that the therapist bears the responsibility for giving way initially and bending towards the client's needs. Later, one of the main goals of therapy may be to try to change the client's style of construing.

Types of construct

In the section above we referred to the way in which constructs lead to varying or unvarying predictions. This is one of the ways in which our constructs control the elements lying within their range. Kelly proposed three further ways in which constructs exert an influence on elements.

1 'A *pre-emptive* construct is one which pre-empts its elements for membership in its own realm exclusively' (**Bannister and Fransella,** 1986, p18; our emphasis). An example of such construing might be, 'he is a stutterer and therefore nothing but a stutterer'. This limits the other ways in which a 'stutterer' may be construed. The person has been classified and cannot belong to any other category. Very few constructs are likely to be used in this way, and if we encounter them in therapy we may have difficulty helping a person change.

2 'A *constellatory* construct is one which fixes the other realm membership of its elements' (**Bannister and Fransella,** 1986, p19; our emphasis). The use of one construct immediately evokes a cluster of others. For example, if this person is a 'stutterer' then he must also be disfluent, anxious about talking, left-handed, intelligent and male. The person has been stereotyped. As therapists we are encouraged to use constellatory constructs when we make a diagnosis. Once we have attached a label it may be difficult to view the client in other ways.

3 A *propositional* construct 'leaves its elements open to construction in all other respects' (**Kelly,** 1955, p155; our emphasis). For example, when we meet a person who stutters, this is only one way of construing him or her, and we will need to find out other things in order to make full sense of this person. To be propositional provides us with an invitation to elaborate our construing. What else do we need to know, if we are to understand the events/people before us? Therefore a propositional view provides us with a spirit of inquiry and the potential to change.

No person uses one mode of construing to the exclusion of others. At different times, and for different purposes, we may use each mode. As therapists, our task is to be aware of the potential for change and the possible obstacles to change in our clients. Even though propositional construing offers room for manoeuvre, the exclusive use of such construing would preclude the ability to home in on the crucial issues in any situation. It is highly likely that we most frequently use the constellatory mode of construing, but, if this does not lead us to make good sense of the issue at hand, being propositional may be helpful. Take, for example, a young child who gives her mother a birthday card she has drawn herself. Mum promptly bursts into tears. To the child, tears signal sadness, pain or distress—a constellation of 'bad' outcomes. At the same time, Mum hugs and kisses her daughter and does not seem sad, in pain or distress. If the child is able to be propositional and ask herself what else Mum's tears might mean, her experiment is likely to be validated and she will learn that she has produced the desired outcome—a happy Mum.

Why people change

(a) Constructs of transition

Kelly proposed a system of diagnostic constructs which are useful for understanding why people change or fail to change. Although the terms may seem familiar, Kelly has defined them in unusual ways. Each dimension has to do with change, and together these dimensions form the emotional content of personal construct theory.

▶ *Anxiety is the awareness that the events with which one is confronted lie mostly outside the range of convenience of one's construct system.*

When a person cannot use their construct system as a basis for making sense of events they experience anxiety. To a person who stutters, listener reactions are a minefield of unknown possibilities, and so all effort is made to try and be fluent. Focusing on the effort to be fluent gives the situation some structure and pulls the unknown back into the known. Because of the intensity of effort involved and the fact that trying not to stutter often precipitates stuttering, the person has no chance to focus on listener reactions and hence may be just as anxious in the next situation.

Anxiety is a source of change. Too much anxiety may be immobilising, but if our anxiety is more circumscribed, we have been offered an opportunity to expand our construing. We may back away sometimes, but at others we accept the challenge and take a leap into the unknown.

▶ *Aggressiveness is the active elaboration of one's perceptual field.*

When we take the plunge and actively experiment and evaluate our construing, we are being aggressive in Kelly's terms. When stuttering clients leave the therapy room and try out a new way of talking, for example stuttering voluntarily, then we can say they are being aggressive. Their experiment does not always come off, but they are to be commended for trying to extend and elaborate their construing. Aggressiveness is therefore the actual substance of change in personal construct theory terms.

▶ *Threat is the awareness of an imminent comprehensive change in one's core structures.*

When our major ways of making sense of the world in which we live are invalidated, we will feel threatened, because, if we accept the invalidation, we are going to have to engage in major reconstruction. For example, a client who seeks therapy may feel very threatened when the therapist says that 'a cure' is possible. Spouses may feel threatened when their husbands or wives go away to do an intensive course. What will they be like when they come back? Will they be very different? A person who has done well in therapy may feel very threatened if perchance she meets someone from her previous therapy group on the street. Can she maintain fluency if the other person stutters? Going back to work after an intensive course might evoke threat for clients. Will they be viewed as 'failures' if they stutter after having therapy? What will colleagues expect of them?

The knowledge that therapy can be threatening for a client leaves therapists with the task of assessing ways of minimising the threats.

Breaking down change into small, manageable steps and making sure that clients are able to make sense of the process are ways of containing the risks of change.

▶ **Guilt is the awareness of dislodgement of the self from one's core role structure.**

Core role constructs are those that capture the essence of self. When we find ourselves doing important things that violate our sense of self, we experience dislodgement. A pacifist would experience guilt in Kellian terms if he sensed he could be violent. Parents of a child who stutters might experience guilt. If they say of themselves, 'We are not the sort of parents whose children have problems' they will feel guilty whenever their child stutters. Such parents might ignore the stuttering, and possibly the child in the process, in their effort not to feel guilty. But guilt is not reserved only for dislodgement in a negative direction from our core role. A person who stutters might experience guilt when speaking fluently. A woman who achieves a powerful position at work may feel guilty if she defines herself as a mother and wife first.

Therapy may easily dislodge clients from their core role. It may be that this is the only way to produce change. Acknowledgement of this possibility and providing clients with alternative ways of construing themselves may make the process of change bearable.

▶ **Hostility is the continued effort to extort validational evidence in favour of a type of social prediction which has already been recognised as a failure.**

We are likely to become hostile when we cannot afford to be wrong; when our investment in a particular outcome of an experiment is greater than our curiosity. If we were to accept that our assumptions were inappropriate, we would be faced with the task of trying again in a different way. This might imply that we have to abandon important structures and leave ourselves vulnerable, and we are likely to become hostile. For example, therapists are frequently hostile when they teach the same technique to clients who have previously failed to improve. It is as if the therapist says to herself, 'I know this technique will work. Even if I have to get Joe to slow down and say one-word utterances for the rest of his life, I will prove that it does'.

Hostility preserves structure. It means that, for the moment, we do not have to face the difficulties of changing. Although it is relatively easy to recognise, it is not until we know what prediction has failed that we can truly understand hostility in another person.

All the constructs of transition have important therapeutic implications. They explain both why we may change and why we may not. Although described under discrete headings, the constructs of transition often merge to produce a process of change. Aggressiveness pushes us forward into new territory: hostility holds us back from the edge.

(b) Conditions that lead to change

If we can provide clients with *fresh elements* to construe there is a likelihood that, as these are successively construed, changes in both content and structure of their systems will ensue. For example, during desensitisation, clients may be asked to conduct a survey on attitudes to stuttering. The answers from the public, whether positive or negative, provide new and varied ways of thinking about stuttering. As clients absorb the evidence it is likely that they will have to form new constructs, or modify old ones.

Where clients are prepared to experiment and test out the grounds on which they make predictions, change is likely to follow. A task such as keeping eye contact while speaking may help clients to understand more about the way listeners react to stuttering. In order to evaluate the results of experiments, validating data is required. The implication of this is that, as therapists, we must have a good notion of the sources of validation available to clients before we send them out with a new experiment tucked up their sleeves. Role playing in therapy, giving the client and therapist the chance to play both parts, is a useful way of trying out new constructs and allowing both parties to match the prediction to the outcome: in other words, to seek validational evidence before taking the experiment outside.

Certainly in the early stages of therapy, the therapist may be the sole provider of validation for the client. Often the therapist can unwittingly be drawn into colluding with the client's constructions of events, thus blocking change. A client may talk of consistently bad reactions to stuttering from one particular colleague at work. In an effort to show empathy, the therapist may agree that the colleague's behaviour is despicable, validating the client's construction of events. Then the client describes another person who reacts badly to stuttering, and the therapist may find it difficult to react differently, and so again confirms the client's view of listeners. The aim in therapy is to help the client reconstrue role relationships with others, but by validating the client's ways of understanding others the therapist may block the process of change. As Kelly puts it, we need to give the right answers to the right questions and this involves a careful understanding of what constructs the client is seeking to have validated.

(c) Conditions which block change

When the implications of change are threatening to the superordinate constructs in the person's system they may be unable to accept the evidence with which they are confronted. Suppose we provide a client with fresh elements to construe, such as described previously, where we asked clients to conduct a survey on attitudes to stuttering. The client discovers that people are less fussed about stuttering than predicted. Although this is pleasantly surprising on one level, the client is confronted with unpleasant evidence at another level. For all of his life the client may have postponed doing things until he achieved some form of fluency. All choices have been governed by these more superordinate role expectations. If he is to accept the results of the survey a major way of structuring his life will have been invalidated. Such a client may resort to hostility and may say, 'People were too afraid to tell us the truth' or 'If a fluent speaker had asked the questions, the answers would have been different'.

Another obstacle to change occurs when clients become preoccupied with old material. The constructs which were useful in the past have no predictive efficiency in the present. Sessions become repetitive and the client seems to be making no headway. An example of this occurred in sessions with a client called Rob. Before he left home, he developed a close relationship with a girl-friend he had known at school. When this relationship ended, he was left without a source of validation for the kind, caring, loving part of his life. He would go back over the fact in every session that everything would be all right if he had a girl-friend. It became apparent that he construed his ex-girl-friend and mother in similar terms. He had replaced one dependency relationship with another, and had lost both—one by moving far away from home and growing up, and the other by the break-up of the relationship. He presented the lack of a girl-friend as the only obstacle to change. When asked to look at his dependency needs and how they might be validated elsewhere, he would hark back to his ex-girl-friend. He seemed unable to apply any of the constructs around that relationship to any of his current women friends; nor was he inclined to develop new ways of construing them.

Dealing with such a client is not easy. The client has to agree to co-operate and to pack away the old constructs for the time being, while seeking new ways of construing. The therapist may have to invalidate the old constructs, to render them inoperative. The client may resort to hostile behaviour in order to protect self against impending change, and so therapy may need to proceed slowly and carefully, taking account of the risks of change.

Unless the client has a 'laboratory' in which to test out new constructs, it is unlikely that any will be formed. An extremely isolated client, who is unemployed and lives alone, will find it difficult to test new constructs about role relationships in the absence of friends or some context in which to change. The therapy room provides only a limited forum for experimentation, but part of the therapy process may need to involve setting up some contexts in which further experimentation may take place. An example of such a client was Terry, who lived just such an isolated existence. After many tasks of construing television characters and general 'people watching' we encouraged Terry to join the Association for Stammerers. This provided him with a forum in which to try out new ways of relating to others, limiting the threats because the others also stuttered.

Facilitating change

Change is unlikely to occur in any form unless constructs are tested. Kelly's view of the person-as-scientist is relevant to this discussion. As in scientific research, the starting-point is to gain an understanding of the person's theories about people and events. Kelly names this process 'controlled elaboration'. The exploratory procedures described in *chapter two* are all examples of controlled elaboration, as is the structured conversation used to discover the client's view of the problem. These procedures provide the therapist with information about the content, structure, process and style of construing.

The main tool of change is the process of experimentation which may help to define or extend the person's construct system, so that the person no longer feels stuck. When ready, the client is invited to make specific predictions. The therapist may ask, 'What would your boss do if . . .? What would he not do? What other possibilities are there?' Then the client can be encouraged to check the predictions made during the session. Kelly believes that testing the prediction becomes irresistible after a while. After all, the client has a structure within which to experiment.

Other ways of encouraging active experimentation involve asking the client to interpret others' outlooks. With a client who uses two major constructs, *likes me–does not like me; respects me–does not respect me* for every encounter, no matter how trivial, the therapist may ask, 'What do you think I focus on when I buy a bus ticket?' Because this client was able to construe the therapist reasonably well, he volunteered, 'You would probably focus on getting a ticket, getting the correct money and that sort of thing'. The therapist asked, 'As opposed to . . .?' and the client replied, 'Focusing on feelings and how other people were seeing you'. The client was invited to enact such a transaction and try on the therapist's construct for size. This will lead on to experimenting outside as the client develops new ways of separating 'important personal' events from 'unimportant impersonal' ones.

All of these procedures and others are described in more detail in the remaining chapters. In this chapter we have focused on both the vocabulary and the process of change in personal construct theory terms. How these ideas are applied and indications for their use form the basis of the rest of this book.

Conclusion

The goal of therapy is to facilitate change, not to specify a particular outcome. When we give a person a gift of money, it is a more generous gift if we encourage them to spend it in any way they choose. So it is in stuttering therapy. As therapists we would be hostile if fluency and nothing but fluency was the only satisfactory outcome of therapy. To approach therapy with the proposition, 'Let us see how we can enable this person to change to their own satisfaction', offers a rich variety of opportunities for both therapist and client.

UNDERSTANDING THE FAMILY AND CHILD

CHAPTER 4
UNDERSTANDING THE FAMILY AND CHILD

Introduction

In this chapter we consider a wide range of information that may help the therapist make sense of a child's stuttering. As a general rule, the younger the child and the milder the stutter, the less information required and the more likely we are to work with the parents rather than the child. As stuttering develops, and so influences the child's psychological development, so we are more likely to include the child in the initial exploration and therapy.

There are two important and interrelated issues that need to be considered, before selecting exploratory procedures.

1 Who is the client? Is it the child, the mother, the parents or the family?
2 Do we work directly with the child's behaviour or do we change the view of the problem so that a new set of alternatives becomes available?

These two possibilities were termed 'first order change' and 'second order change' by **Watzlawick *et al.*** (1974). All speech techniques aim for first order change while work on altering the parent's construing of the child and the problem aims for second order change. Once we have decided with whom we wish to work, and the order of change to aim for, we can begin to select appropriate procedures. We would like to make some general points before we describe the exploratory procedures:

■ Sessions will need to be at least an hour long.

■ We aim to see the parents and child together on the first meeting, so that we can get a sense of how they interact and deal with the communication problem.

■ Exploration and therapy are not two discrete phases: many of the procedures described in this chapter will trigger the process of change.

■ Exploratory sessions aim at being a structured conversation rather than an interview. When clients are engaged in the process of understanding and clarifying the problem they are more likely to find the experience useful. It is important that parents leave the session with some positive feelings, not drained by endless questions.

■ People should not feel compelled to answer questions when they wish to remain silent.

■ For us, the initial exploration is a phase of hypothesis making and testing and this is what guides our lines of approach and the selection of questions. Standard questionnaires can alienate clients and stop us exploring important areas.

The chapter is divided into two main sections: first we consider the family, then the child. Within each section different approaches to exploring the meaning of stuttering are described. Decisions concerning which parts to use with any particular client will depend upon the therapist's theoretical position and skills, as well as what seems appropriate to the client and possible within available resources.

The family

(a) The role of the parents in therapy

There is considerable controversy surrounding the whole issue of the parents' role in the development of stuttering. Their involvement in speech therapy is equally controversial. The extreme positions are that:

1 Therapy should be with the parents, and the focus upon their responses to stuttering rather than the stuttering itself (**Clifford and Watson**, 1987).
2 It is difficult to change parents' behaviour and there is no proof that it influences the child's fluency; therefore
    . . . a more suitable strategy for treating stuttering in young children is to directly teach them to produce fluent, non-stuttered speech no matter what is going on in their natural environment. (**Costello**, 1983, p73)

Both these views lack hard evidence to support them and the therapist is left to decide for herself which view she subscribes to or whether she will play it safe and use an approach that combines working with the parents with some direct work on the child's expressive speech. It is our belief that work with parents is important. Not only has our work with parents led to reductions in disfluency, but also many of the adults whom we have talked with think that their parents' ignorance and fear played a major role in the development of their stuttering problem. In our experience many adults have never spoken with their parents openly and easily about stuttering and do not recall doing so as children. When they do manage to broach the subject they often find their parents are ill-informed about stuttering and feel guilty and ashamed of the problem.

(b) Our justification for working with the parents of the referred child

- The child's communication skills develop within the context of the family and so the family interaction has a profound effect on how these skills develop;
- The major part of the child's communication with adults occurs within the family. Usually talking to adults is more difficult for the child than talking to peers;
- The significance that the problem has for the family as a whole and for each member personally can only be understood by meeting them all. This should help to identify how the problem with speaking fits into the family's structure and construing;
- Observation of patterns of interaction and the quality of communication will identify some of the causal and maintaining factors.

We support the position taken by **Clezy** (1979) when she argues that:

1 the notion of the therapist 'curing' the child is misguided;
2 the mother's inclusion in therapy improves the interaction between mother and child;
3 the mother fulfils the role of clinical aid with greater motivation and more time than can ever be provided by the health service;

4 the mother acquires a knowledge of processes important to the development of children as a whole which will benefit her subsequent children as well as others that she has contact with.

We would argue that both parents may have a contribution to make to therapy.

Although Clezy was discussing language and phonological problems, her comments are relevant to the problem of stuttering. In addition, she recognises that therapists are often called upon to provide counselling on other areas of child development. We argue that the scope of the therapist should, where possible, be extended to include not only the family, but also the everyday child care problems that many parents struggle with.

Our justification for taking this broader view of children is that verbal communication occurs in every situation throughout the normal day. Problems with feeding, sleeping, tantrums and the rest have an influence upon the communication between parents and child. When parents feel that they are not coping or that their child is becoming too demanding they will have difficulty in attending to the child's communication needs. We can take this argument further and hypothesise that in some cases the disfluent speech is the result of the strain that the family is feeling. When the therapist feels unable to extend her role in this way, through lack of training and experience, then we would suggest working with a health visitor or other colleague.

A further issue to consider concerns the relationship between different behaviours. In personal construct theory a person's behaviour is considered from the point of view of its function for the individual. For example, it may be that a child's refusal to eat and his disfluent speech are alike in that they both occur when the child feels invalidated. If we look at different behaviours and seek out similarities and differences we may be surprised at the way that seemingly different behaviours fit together. By attributing responsibility for different problems to different professionals, a holistic view of the child may be lost. The *patterns of behaviour* may be missed and hence we may fail to understand why the child behaves as he does.

When attempting to understand a child's speaking problem, it is as if we need to put on a different set of glasses to explore each aspect of the child and his family. At the end the task is to sort these different perceptions into a coherent pattern that will then indicate the next step in therapy. It is difficult to wear more than one pair of glasses at a time and if the focus is on the interaction and communication within the family, it may be impossible to assess the child's level of language skill simultaneously. Likewise, while assessing the child's language it may be difficult to attend adequately to the interaction patterns.

The rest of the chapter is written with the image of 'different glasses' very much in mind. As the therapist tests a hypothesis, the client will be viewed in a particular way. If the hypothesis is disproved another approach can be taken. The following example may help to illustrate this. At the beginning of the session the child may say very little and be unintelligible to the therapist. The therapist considers the possibility of a language-based problem. As the session develops it is noticed that the father interacts very little with the child and that the mother speaks for the child. This raises the hypotheses that the mother and child are excluding the father and that the mother is trying to protect the child, either from being misunderstood by the father or from stuttering. If the child then talks freely and in an age-appropriate manner while playing with a sibling, the initial hypothesis is questioned. As the session develops the parents may relax and the father take a more active role with the child and so the second hypothesis requires some revision. If we encourage the family to interact our hypotheses will be tested. If, however, we just listen to the parents' version of things we may fail to test our hypotheses and hence misunderstand the problem.

The questions we ask will influence the data that we acquire and so, initially, it is helpful to consider stuttering in a relatively loose manner. This should help us to be open to a variety of possibilities; then as we collect information we can tighten our construing of the particular problems raised and arrive at some therapeutic strategies.

We suggest that the length of time spent on understanding the problem should be determined by the needs of the client and not imposed *a priori*. It is most unlikely that such an exploration will take as long as it takes to treat an adult who stutters. Time spent with the child and family represents a good investment.

(c) Understanding the family

Whenever possible we recommend that two therapists be involved in the exploratory sessions. It is extremely difficult to work with a family and pick up everything. A therapist on her own can get caught up in the family's view of things and lose her perspective. A colleague observing, either in the room or behind a mirror, can help by providing another account. Video recordings of the session will also help.

(i) Family tree or genogram

The construction of a family tree is an excellent way of inviting the family to introduce themselves to the therapist. Drawing a tree while the family provides the information moves the focus away from the child and on to where the child comes from and currently lives. It is usual to refer to three generations, including the grandparents. Previous marriages and children are recorded and the therapist may wish to note those who have maintained close contact with the family. Some practice is required before drawing a client's tree since they are often quite complicated, with death, divorce, additional children, miscarriage and so on all needing to be recorded and vying for space on the paper. Using large sheets of paper is helpful and also enables the family members to see the tree as it develops. When possible, all members of the family may be included in the task. In this way the therapist communicates her interest in everyone's views. The whole exercise will be more useful if the drawing of the tree is undertaken as a way of learning about the family and members' differing views of it. Conversations about the contributions that different family members make, and the special rela-tionships that exist, help the family tree to come alive. Sometimes a family photograph album can be used to encourage discussion about the different members of the family. An example of a simple family tree is given below.

(ii) Family life cycle

The concept of the family life cycle recognises the family as an evolving and developing unit. At each stage of the cycle the different generations of the family have different but interrelated roles. **Dare** (1979) suggests the following phases: babyhood; toddler; Oedipal; school entry; pre-adolescence and adolescence; young adulthood; courtship and marriage; pregnancy and babyhood-parental; mid-life; old age. When Dare considers the school entry phase, he shows the interrelationships as follows:

Figure 4.1 A family tree

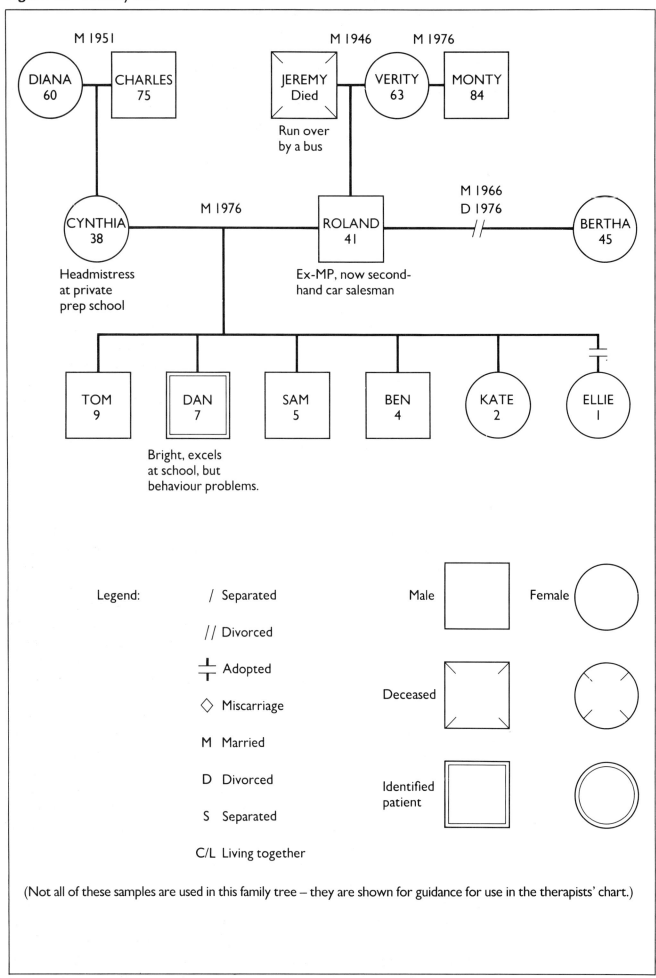

Legend:
/ Separated

// Divorced

┴┬ Adopted

◇ Miscarriage

M Married

D Divorced

S Separated

C/L Living together

Male

Female

Deceased

Identified patient

(Not all of these samples are used in this family tree – they are shown for guidance for use in the therapists' chart.)

Source: The symbols are from **Barker P,** *Basic Family Therapy,* Collins, London, 1986.

- The tasks for the **child** of school age are:
  Accept care from adult other than parents.
  Share caring adult with classmates.
  Enjoy and use peers for self-development.
  Discover particular interests and become able to work.

- The **parents'** role in the world is more defined and established and they have increasing authority. Their parenting tasks are:
  Accept [child's] *ability to separate and allow closeness to peers and to teachers;*
  Encourage [child's] *interests, even when different from the family.*

- The **grandparents** can:
  Provide holiday time away from parents.
  Act as additional identifactory adults. **Dare** (pp 142–3)

Considering the family at their current stage in the life cycle can help to identify the major tasks that concern each individual. Their ability to develop as the particular stage demands can be assessed. Help can be directed towards this development when it is failing to occur. For example, the child's fear of school and of talking to teachers may well be related to the parents' inability to allow the child to develop independence. The grandparents may also be playing a part by providing constant interference rather than occasional support. Consideration of the family life cycle is not a sufficient assessment, but rather a useful framework within which to explore the current issues for the family. When considered along with the family tree, a picture unfolds of the family, past, present and anticipating the future.

(iii) The family construct system

Much of the work on family construct systems is being developed by **Procter** (1985a). He works as a family therapist using techniques and ideas from brief therapy. However he avoids the 'trap of eclecticism' (p1, 1986) by using personal construct theory as his superordinate or umbrella framework and so uses a variety of techniques with a Kellian purpose. The family construct system has the features of a personal construct system but in addition relies upon members of the family interacting with each other and hence validating or invalidating each individual's perceptions of the shared system. For example, the 'irresponsible' teenager feels that his mother is being unfair and does not understand him when she complains and tells him to stay in. He protests by going out. This type of interaction tends to escalate in a symmetrical fashion; that is, the more the mother complains the more the boy goes out, so the more cause for complaint the mother has and so on. Each person's construing of the other is validated by this type of escalation which makes it difficult to stop. Other family members are likely to be drawn in and their negative construction of the 'problem' person will also be validated. One can think of a similar pattern that may exist with a younger, disfluent child (see *Figure 4.2* overleaf).

If disfluent speech has particularly negative implications for one or both of the parents their behaviour in response to the hesitations may confuse and alarm the child further. For example, if one of them stutters or if the mother found it hard to construe the needs of her pre-verbal infant, she may be especially threatened by any problems with spoken communication. Many infants, especially the first-born, fail to conform to parental expectations. The discovery of just how unpredictable small babies can be increases the sense of novelty and challenge for some parents and catapults others into

Figure 4.2 Cycle of parent–child interaction

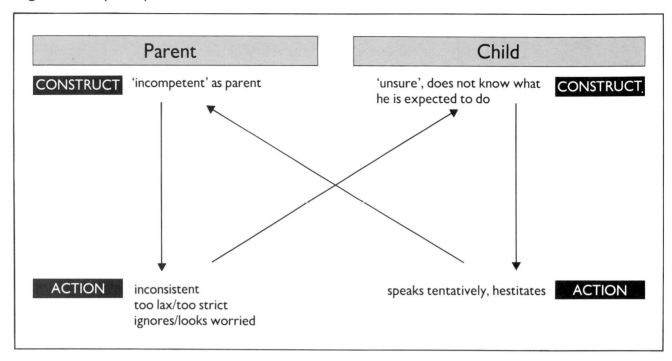

chaos. This latter group seems to be more disturbed by disfluent speech and needs more counselling than the former group.

When considering family construct systems we must remember that each new baby has an effect on the system as they validate or invalidate different predictions. There will be constructs from the families of origin of both parents as well as the influences of current thinking concerning childcare. Many of the constructs in the parents' personal systems will include the family in their range of convenience. As the child's system develops, so his input into the family system may change it. Presumably a stable family is able to retain the superordinate family structure while accommodating the influences of outside lives, the past and so on. A crisis is likely to occur when the superordinate constructs within the family system are threatened.

(iv) How do we get to know the family construct system?

It is necessary to meet the family and to listen, not so much to the detailed content of what has occurred, but rather to the different ways in which family members talk about their significant experiences. We attempt to tune in to the language that they use and listen for constructs. Labelling the implicit ends of constructs and exposing the different and idiosyncratic dichotomies that family members hold can go a long way towards increasing mutual understanding. For example, different family members may use the word 'boring', but each attaches a different meaning which becomes clear when the other end of the construct is verbalised:

Boring–'makes me feel good'
Boring–'easy'
Boring–'exciting'
Boring–'allowed to choose for myself'

It is stretching the point to call the negative end 'boring' in each case, but the idea is to show how shades of meaning can be quite different for different family members and that when these are not discussed openly misunderstandings and bad feelings are likely to arise. As the meanings of different constructs are negotiated so the individual members become better able to construe each other's construction processes (play a role in relation to each other). **Procter** (1986) describes a strategy for exploring the meanings of family constructs that not only provides information, but also clarifies things for the family. If the word 'noisy' seems relevant then each member of the family is given the chance to say whom they think is the most 'noisy'. This should generate discussion that will help to clarify the meaning that the construct has for family members. This type of questioning is rather like completing a live family grid, ranking elements rather than rating them. Quite young children can be included in this sort of discussion although they may prefer to use miniature people or some other visual means.

This discussion of similarities and differences can also provide information about:

1 The family's ability to tolerate differences and also their methods of dealing with disagreement;
2 Alliances within the family;
3 Who, if anyone, must ultimately speak for the family;
4 The degree of respect that family members have for each other's contributions.

When the discussion moves between construing and behaviour, family members are encouraged to construe each others' behaviour in different ways. If the mother complains about the child being too noisy and excitable, then initially these constructs can be explored and later the different reasons for behaving in this way can be considered. If the mother grew up in a home where noise signalled an angry father perhaps she and her mother learnt to make themselves scarce at such times. The link between noise and her feelings when her father was angry will be strong. Although her child's noisiness is obviously quite different her responses may still be linked to the earlier, frequently validated construction. Construing noisiness from her child's point of view will relieve her of considerable pain as well as enable her to behave more appropriately. Perhaps if she can join in the noisy game and then help move her child towards some other activity both would benefit.

There are further questions that **Procter** (1985a) suggests will help the therapist understand the family construct system:

- Whom does he take after more, his mother or his father?
- Whom is he closer to?
- In what way are they different/similar?
- What makes you say that he gets nervous/confident?

This 'live grid' questioning satisfies the need within family therapy and construct therapy to attend to processes and not merely the cataloguing of events. A therapist who encourages a family to negotiate shared meanings moves from the safety of observation into the somewhat threatening waters of playing a role in relation to the family. As the therapist begins to construe the family system so the presenting problems begin to make sense.

The family view of the problem is also of interest. Do they see stuttering as a sort of illness requiring treatment or do they see it as some sort of badness? Quite often one hears the suggestion that it is caused by laziness, and gradually it becomes apparent that laziness is subsumed under a *good–bad* construct. When the stuttering is viewed as an illness it is likely that physical remedies have been tried, for example, change of diet or sleeping habits.

The solutions that the family have tried may well be playing a part in the maintenance of the problem and so it is important to find out about these. The parents can be asked what they do when the child stutters, how the child responds and then what they do in return. In this way a picture can be constructed of the sequences of events around stuttering. Observation of the family should also provide information about the solutions that they try.

If we take the view that in some way stuttering makes sense to the family group, we need to understand its meaning and effects. The family can be asked how things have changed since the child started stuttering and how things would be different if he stopped. If the parents were not concerned about the child's speaking, where would they be directing their energies?

We can also find out if the family are inclined to polarise the different members. In our experience the stuttering child is often viewed quite negatively, with another sibling being seen as the 'good' opposite. This may be most apparent when a male stuttering child has a fluent sister. The sister is seen as a confident, competent and fluent child who presents the parents with few problems, while the stuttering child is considered nervous, incompetent, and generally difficult. One problem with this sort of polarisation is that it tends to escalate; the 'good' child seems even better in relation to the 'bad' child and as she gets 'better' so he gets 'worse'. Other people may contribute to this also: teachers may polarise the two children, as may grandparents and so on. The stuttering child is offered fewer and fewer contexts in which to redeem himself and the fluent child is encouraged to excel in more and more ways. Before long this process becomes a problem for everyone and especially the children, neither of whom can relinquish their positions.

(d) Observation of family interaction and communication

In this section we consider how speech therapists view family interaction. The most obvious differences between speech and family therapists is that the former focus more narrowly upon the interactions around speaking, and they aim to teach skills that produce first order change. Another difference lies in the controversy that surrounds the importance of family interaction. For family therapists there is no doubt about the importance of patterns of interaction: the debate is centred around how best to change them. Speech therapists debate whether or not such patterns are important, and whether they are amenable to change.

Egolf *et al.* (1972) suggest that stuttering represents the child's adjustment to his environment and that it is the parents' parallel adjustment that maintains the stuttering. In this sense 'the dyad is in equilibrium' (p222). Their assessment aims to identify the maintaining behaviours and therapy aims to establish a new equilibrium by changing the behaviour of both child and parent(s). For example, if the parent was an inattentive and critical listener then the therapist would be attentive and accepting. Thus the therapist models the desired parental behaviour while encouraging fluency by appropriate direct means. Once fluency is established the parent attempts the alternative listening behaviour. Video-recordings are used to study parent—child interaction and later to assess the degree of change. Parents are shown the initial recording and invited to comment on how they have changed.

Another approach is to study a number of families and look for recurring behaviours that appear to disrupt communication and then to look for these in subsequent families. This approach is suggested by **Riley and Riley** (1979, 1983) in their Component Model. The disruptive behaviours that they observed in 53 per cent of their population were:

1 Conversations that were too rapidly paced;

2 Insufficient silent periods for the child who stutters to organize his thoughts;

3 Interrupting the child during his attempts to communicate;

4 Acting rushed while waiting for the child to respond. (1983, p53)

Prins (1983) agrees that these behaviours are likely to produce disfluency in a child at risk. In addition he identifies the following as creative of problems: complex adult speech; verbal 'teaching'; questions that require complex answers from the child and a competitive speaking environment.

Gregory (1985) recommends the analysis of interaction as well as a discussion to identify general and specific pressures. The specific behaviours that he lists are similar to those above, but he makes some additional points: for example, filling in words; finishing the child's statement; guessing what the child is about to say; constant correction of the child's verbal and non-verbal behaviour; failure to respond to the content of the child's speech; frequent changes in topic.

When examining the lists cited above, the importance of not separating disfluency from other communication problems becomes clear. The child who is experiencing difficulty in developing the required skills to ensure fluent and comfortable speaking is as sensitive to communication variables as any other young child. Unfortunately it is usual in the speech pathology literature to separate the different types of communication problems. Implications of research in one area of disability are seldom linked to other problems. A recent exception to this is 'A Pragmatic Study of Child Disfluency' (**Pollack et al.**, 1986). This single case-study looked at conversational breakdowns, repairs and resolution strategies that occurred during a conversation between a mother and her 3-year 9-month-old daughter, who had been diagnosed as stuttering. The mother opted for highly structured activities and the daughter's stuttering occurred when she initiated a departure from her mother's design. The authors suggest that the child was attempting to gain some control over the situation. Perhaps the stuttering was an indication of how difficult it was for the child to gain control in the face of the mother's desire to 'teach' her child. It is interesting that we have already mentioned 'verbal teaching' (see Prins above) as a possible fluency disruptor. It seems likely that further work done on language use will have relevance to our understanding of stuttering.

Interaction checklists can be derived from the literature and may provide a useful guide for therapists. It is important that the child's responses are also recorded since it is the factors that lead to disfluency or distress that are of particular interest to us. We must be wary when using such lists that we do not impose our own high standards on our clients. Probably we can all think of families where everyone talks loudly and quickly at the same time, rarely listening and with the added distractions of television, radio, cats and dogs, and their children all develop fluent, intelligible and age-appropriate communication. This brings us back once more to the importance of understanding personal meanings and not just cataloguing behaviours or observed events.

(e) General environmental factors

The same controversy exists when we consider general environmental factors as was seen with specific communication factors. If we forget stuttering for a moment and think of problem behaviours as a symptom of family disfunction, then quite obviously we are justified in considering the ways different members experience the family group. Although the value of viewing stuttering as a family symptom has not been assessed, the practice of seeing the child in the context of the family is gaining acceptance. Some of the factors that the proponents of this view have identified are listed below. **Prins** (1983, p28) points to the following general sources of environmental stress and uncertainty:

a. Erratic planning and conduct of routine daily activities including meals and bedtime.
b. Activity schedules that create unsettling time pressures.
c. Continuing, unpredictable changes in the makeup of the 'family' constellation, including relatives and visitors who sometimes live in the home, parental absences, etc.
d. Behavioural demands the child is unable to meet.
e. Insufficient time spent alone with the child and in attending to his individual needs.

Rustin and Cook (1983) also consider uncertainty or lack of predictability to be a problem. They take an essentially behavioural view of the problem and value consistent reinforcement. They stress the importance of reinforcement for the parents and therefore the necessity of moving their focus away from stuttering and onto fluent speaking. They have found that a focus on speaking behaviour alone is limiting and cite an example of a feeding problem that was solved with benefit to both child and mother. In assessment they look for problem-solving strategies since 'good problem-solvers tend to show better social adjustment when dealing with these problems [that is, conflict situations] than those with limited abilities in this area'.

Riley and Riley (1983, p53) found that half their sample of parents had high expectations of their children: 'verbally or attitudinally, parents demanded "perfection" academically, behaviourally, and developmentally'. In their assessment 89 per cent of the children had high expectations and wished to be better than their peer group. When these high standards are applied to speaking performance both parents and child may focus upon the disfluencies. **Sheehan** (1975) talked about the importance of balancing the demands that are made of the child with the supports that he receives. This idea of a *demand—support* ratio is helpful when evaluating how the child is coping with pressures. The idea of support can be extended to include not only what the parents provide, but also what the child's current level of development makes possible. For example, being expected to talk in sentences and answer questions may not have been a problem when the first-born daughter was two-and-a-half but might be unrealistic for the second-born son at the same age. The child may have developed their own set of priorities and when these fail to coincide with those of the parents, problems can arise.

Understanding the significance that different behaviours have for the family is an important prerequisite to suggesting changes. This can be illustrated by an example from a mothers' study group (**Hayhow**, 1986). The topic of discussion was sibling fights and the strategy of leaving them to it had been tried. One mother was pleased that her refusal to become involved had led her children to the realisation that fighting did not solve problems. This seemed to her more important than the bloody nose that the smaller one acquired in the process. Another mother was horrified that the fight should have been allowed to progress this far. She had a very strong opposition to any form of physical violence and in addition the provision of protection was an important aspect of her role as mother.

This example serves to illustrate the importance of understanding the

60

construing behind an event. We should not attempt to make all families orderly, predictable and child-centred, but rather try to identify those areas that are generating problems and then attempt to understand how they fit into the family view of life. Only then should we make suggestions or, better still, provide a context in which creative thinking can occur so that the parents may decide for themselves how to go about making some changes. Many of the families that we have worked with over the years do have problems of a general nature. However there have been very few where the family was disfunctioning sufficiently severely to indicate referral.

The child

Throughout the time spent getting to know the family we also need to listen to the child. It is likely that an impression will have been gained as to the severity of the stuttering. The age-appropriateness of the child's language skills will have been noted; however, it is still desirable to assess them more formally if there is any doubt. The reported incidence of speech and language problems among disfluent children varies from one piece of research to the next, but there is increasing evidence to suggest that at least 50 per cent will have, or have had, some problem (for example, **Blood and Seider**, 1981; **Gregory**, 1985).

(a) Assessment of the child's disfluency

First, we shall consider the nature and extent of the young child's disfluencies. We can view the therapist's role as differentiating between children at risk of developing chronic stuttering and those less at risk. We are not able to predict with certainty which children will stop stuttering spontaneously.

There is agreement that sound and syllable repetitions are not a regular feature of normal disfluency, whereas word and phrase repetitions are (for example, **Wexler and Mysak**, 1982; **Stournaras**, 1983). In an earlier review of the literature, **Hayhow** (1983) found that the number of times a normally developing child repeated part of a word rarely exceeded one repetition on each occurrence.

Stournaras (1983) found that his sample was more disfluent when speaking in front of the nursery or kindergarten group and when engaged in conversation with a researcher, than in a free-play situation. However the nature of their disfluencies did not change, only the quantity. We can conclude that most children are sensitive to communicative stress but that this does not lead inevitably to syllable repetitions. Only a small group of children will demonstrate multiple repetitions of parts of words when subjected to communicative stress.

The influence of grammatical complexity upon fluency is frequently debated and currently one view is that 'pre-schoolers cannot be treated as a homogeneous group when examining the relationship between language and disfluency behaviours' (**Gordon et al.**, 1986). Their sample were more fluent when imitating linguistically complex material than when the same material was modelled. If stuttering children respond similarly, and we assume that they will, then assessment should include modelled production of linguistically complex material.

Another important aspect of normal disfluency is the way that it changes over time. **DeJoy and Gregory** (1985) compared two groups of thirty non-stuttering boys, with mean ages of three-and-a-half years and five years. They suggest that as children approach school age there is a reduction in the number of repetitions, incomplete phrases and dysrhythmic phonations. Interjections and ungrammatical pauses did not significantly reduce with age and these have been identified as characteristic of adult speech (**Goldman-Eisler**, 1968). Another interesting finding from the DeJoy and Gregory study is that part-word repetitions and dysrhythmic phonations, while apparently independent variables in young children, correlate significantly in the older group. **Wexler and Mysak** (1982) have suggested that these two disfluency types reflect a 'motor factor', and therefore, a five-year-old whose speech still contains these disfluencies must be considered at risk of developing stuttering even when there is no sign of struggle or awareness. It is unlikely that parents will be able to provide detailed descriptions of the child's disfluencies at different ages, but many will have noticed some changes. We must try to assess whether these changes seem to reflect increased skilfulness with verbal expression or whether they suggest increasing difficulty in finishing words.

The frequency of disfluencies can be recorded but there is conflicting evidence regarding what is normal. The table below shows the levels of disfluency found by various researchers for different age groups of non-stuttering children.

Table 4.1   Levels of disfluency in normal speaking children

Authors	Gender	2 years % disfl. SD	3 years % disfl. SD	4 years % disfl. SD	5 years % disfl. SD	6 years % disfl. SD
Yairi (1981)	Boys Girls	7.95 6.39 5.24 3.35				
Wexler & Mysak (1982)	Boys	14.6		9.1 3.2		9.1 4.1
DeJoy & Gregory (1985)	Boys		11.4 4.62		9.3 3.31	

In all the studies the standard deviation is relatively large, which indicates that there is considerable individual variation. Only one study had girl subjects, so we cannot generalise any sex differences. Although we cannot identify at what level disfluency becomes abnormally high we can average the above estimates of disfluency and arrive at 10.5 per cent. We would expect a higher level of fluency when the content is familiar and the listener well-known and liked. As a general guideline, when part-word repetitions are more common than one per hundred words and the overall frequency of disfluencies exceeds 10 per cent there is some cause for concern.

Another important area for investigation concerns the child's handling of disfluency. Any sign of struggle or tension warrants concern. There are many stories of children who have struggled with speaking for a few weeks and then have never re-experienced this difficulty. However struggle is such a basic feature of stuttering that we must take it as a serious indication that speaking has ceased to be a pleasant and easy activity for the child. **Perkins**

(1983) hypothesises that it is involuntary blocking that differentiates the stuttering from the normally disfluent child. He maintains that only those children who experience this involuntary loss of control are seriously at risk of developing life-long stuttering. Those who repeat words or part-words without feeling out of control are likely to become more fluent as they mature. Unfortunately Perkins is not able to tell us how to recognise when the child is out of control. This hypothesis is mentioned because it fits in with clinical observations that there are some children whose stuttering has a compulsive quality from very early on. What is more, the parents of these children are often frightened by the child's difficulties: it is as if they pick up the feelings of panic. Whenever the therapist has evidence that the child feels out of control when stuttering then therapy is indicated.

Summary

In order confidently to diagnose normal disfluency the following criteria should be met in speech samples taken from a variety of situations. Both communicative stress and linguistic complexity should be varied. The parents' descriptions should also be taken into account.

- Part-word repetitions do not generally exceed 1 per cent of words spoken.
- The number of repetitions in each instance of part-word repetition exceed one only occasionally.
- Total disfluencies do not exceed 10–15 per cent.
- As the child approaches school age so the percentage of repetitions, dysrhythmic phonations and incomplete phrases decreases. Interjections and ungrammatical pauses remain much the same so that the overall level of disfluency reduces.
- No signs of tension accompanying the disfluencies.
- There should be no avoidance behaviours.
- The parents agree that these criteria are met.

When there is no doubt that the child is stuttering, speech samples may be obtained to inform the therapist and provide a record. However it is even more difficult to assess a child's progress than it is with adults, since childhood stuttering is episodic. This means that we must rely upon the child, the parents and other concerned adults to inform us of the child's progress. It is unfortunate that fluency in the clinic is no proof of successful treatment. However, when everyone reports that the child no longer stutters and this is still the case two years later, then we can consider final discharge.

(b) Language skills

When a child appears to have good expressive language and comprehension, a screening test is a sufficient assessment. Any areas of deficit can be assessed using the procedures that would be used for a child with a language disability. **Riley and Riley** (1979, 1983) identify some specific difficulties experienced by significant numbers of their stuttering sample. They refer to these as the 'neurologic components' and they are listed here with the percentage of children who demonstrated these difficulties.

A clinical impression gained over the last few years of our work is that there is a subgroup of children who score above their age level on a

Attending disorders	37%
Auditory processing disorders	28%
Sentence formulation disorders	30%
Oral motor disorders	87%

screening test, but who seem to be having difficulty in selecting and retrieving words, structures, and so on. These children were all helped when their parents accepted the children's need to consolidate the skills that they had developed without any pressure to increase either the sophistication of their response or the size of their vocabulary. Although it may sound unacceptably subjective, looking for a balance or imbalance between the skills that the child has, the linguistic demands that are made and the ability to use the skills is more useful than comparison with normative data (see also **Wall and Meyers**, 1984).

(c) Understanding the child

This section considers ways of understanding the child's construing. If we hypothesise that a particular child is using a *stuttering—fluency* construct to make sense of a variety of people and situations, then we can test this by using the techniques in this section, which also provide indicators for therapy. We suggest further exploration when:

1 The child is obviously upset by a relatively mild stutter.
2 The solutions that symptomatic therapy has offered seem to be maintaining the problem. For example, an increase in fluency has led to an increase in fear of stuttering which in turn is increasing either stuttering or avoidance behaviour. Alternatively, the child may be moving backwards and forwards between the two poles of the fluency—stuttering dimension so that changes in speaking are not accompanied by any change in construing.
3 Fluency is clinic-bound and attempts at transfer have failed.
4 Regression has occurred and it is likely that a repetition of previous methods will produce the same pattern of improvement–regression
5 The client shows an interest in *why* he stutters.
6 An adolescent finds it extremely difficult to make socially useful predictions. This may become apparent during preparation for assignment work or earlier if he is asked to describe people whom he knows.

Theoretically there is no reason why we should not elicit constructs and complete a grid with any child of school age. Obviously the methods used must take account of the child's maturational level and interests. However it may be that such extensive exploration of the child's construct system is neither necessary nor appropriate. **Ravenette** (in press) is more interested in the child's constructions than in his constructs. In other words, it is how the child uses his constructs to make sense of everyday events and familiar people that is important. When talking about repertory grids he reminds us that they are 'but one way in which a client's realities may be explored. For many problems, especially with children, there are other productive ways of exploring their constructions'.

Our focus in this section is on observing and conversing with young children. As children develop it is possible to structure conversations more consistently and some methods for doing this are considered in the next section.

(i) Observation and conversation

The way we behave and the choices that we make are governed by our constructs and the ways that we use them. Therefore it should be possible to infer something about a person's construing by watching what they do. This notion was explored by **Beveridge and Brierley** (1982) when they observed nursery-age children. The consistent choices that different children made were noted. The interpretations that they thought appropriate were tested in conversation with the children. There were six constructs that the children seemed to use frequently when having to make decisions about what to do. They were:

my world—not my world
supervised—not supervised
doing—listening
together—alone
home—school
can—can't

They support their selection of constructs with segments of conversations where children verbalise the different constructions. For example the *my world* pole is clearly demonstrated by one child's running commentary as she played outside:

> (As the paddling pool is brought out) . . . I've got a paddling pool . . . I've got pictures on mine . . . I've got a red dress on . . . (on seeing someone skipping) I've got a skipping rope . . . (climbing on the slide) I've not got a slide. (p163)

Two further examples show how *listening* is construed as negative by an active and fairly disruptive boy and as positive by a more passive and anxious girl.

CB: Do you like Mrs Hollingworth telling stories?
Boy: No. I just listen. (p170)

The following child was discussing why she liked stories:

CB: Which do you like best?
Girl: Quiet room (ie story time)
CB: Why is that better?
Girl: Stories.
CB: What about stories?
Girl: I can listen. (p171)

Beveridge and Brierley demonstrate very clearly in this paper that we can learn about children's construing by watching them make decisions and by looking for patterns in their behaviour. As we begin to find children more predictable so we know we are beginning to construe their construction processes.

The way in which a construct system develops is also important if we are to make any judgements about a particular child. Children may talk about a person's behaviour but that does not mean that they are discriminating purely in terms of what people do. Physical descriptions are easier to verbalise than, for example, psychological characteristics. However from an early age children may be linking behaviour and attitudes, and in turn relating these to their own feelings. An example may help to illustrate this. A five-year-old who had not enjoyed his first year in school spoke with some enthusiasm about the teacher he was to have the following year.

Child: I like Mrs X.
Adult: Do you, what do you like about her?
Child: She likes children.
Adult: How do you know she likes children?
Child: She doesn't shout at them all the time.

The child had said before that he did not like the way his current teacher was always shouting and we can see the construction that he places upon this behaviour, which is that teachers who shout do not like children. No wonder he was unhappy! Some two years later, when once more discussing a teacher whom he liked less than a current much-liked teacher, the same child said, 'I didn't like Mrs Y so much because she was always cross and grumbling; Mrs Z likes us and she's happy at school'.

So although it appears that the child is using 'physical' constructs, for example, *shouts—doesn't shout*, they in fact have 'psychological' implications that have been validated over time. A conversation of this type may help us understand the child more than the elicitation of constructs would have done. During conversation we can employ some of the methods discussed in the adult section as well, for example, pyramiding, and the ABC method.

Many of the published procedures for understanding children's construing have been developed by Ravenette in his work as an educational psychologist. He considers that every meeting with a client should be viewed as an opportunity for reconstruction and so the therapist is actively involved in making sense of and developing hypotheses about alternatives throughout an 'assessment' interview. Some of the procedures developed by Ravenette are outlined in the following section.

(ii) Structured conversations

The first two procedures are described in more detail in a chapter by **Ravenette** (1980).

Portrait gallery: This technique is used to elaborate feelings. Two schematic faces are drawn, one to represent a sad boy/girl and the other a happy one. The child is asked to differentiate between the faces and then to say three things about each one. It is important to ask for three things since it seems that children are unable to roll off three glib answers. Asking for three things encourages the child to relate the task to their own feelings. The child is then asked to fill in some blank faces with other feelings and continue in the same way. As an example of this technique, Ravenette presents the following extract from an interview. The child's responses are:

> *Sad:* 1. Naughty, he gets told off. 2. Doesn't get what he wants. 3. Doesn't do as he's told, therefore he gets smacked, therefore he is sad.

> *Happy:* 1. He doesn't get told off all the time. 2. He is good: Mum asks him to do something, he does it, he sets the table. 3. He doesn't want things straight away, he waits, he knows he will get it later. (p47)

Ravenette says of these statements: 'Sadness goes with badness and having to be patient for his needs to be met. Happiness seems not to exist in its own right, but only as a consequence of meeting the demands and values of the parents, or in the absence of sadness' (p48).

The good and the bad of it: This procedure is based upon **Tschudi's** (1977) ABC Model that is discussed in *chapter 2*. Therapist and child agree upon a statement about the current problem, and then what the child would prefer. The child is asked what is 'bad' and 'good' about the first statement and then what is 'good' and 'bad' about the second one. For example:

> I can't talk properly in front of the class.
> The *bad* thing about this is it makes me feel stupid.
> The *good* thing about this is that it gets me out of doing assembly reading.

> I would prefer to talk like everyone else.
> The *good* thing about this is I would feel as clever as everyone else.
> The *bad* thing is that I'd be the same as everyone, nobody would notice me.

This procedure helps us to understand the dilemmas that the problem behaviour holds for the person. The child in the example might benefit from elaborating some of the constructs that he uses to differentiate between people. He is showing the beginnings of the sort of thinking found so often in people who stutter, that is, that the *stuttering—fluency* construct is the most important one for distinguishing between people.

Who are you? (WAY): This technique is described in an earlier paper by **Ravenette** (1977a) and is his adaptation of a procedure used with adult clients. The child is asked a straightforward question:

> Your mother must know you pretty well by now. If I were to ask her what three things she would say were the most important things about you, what would that be?

In this way we are asking the child to tell us what he considers defines his relationships with his mother and then other significant people. We can find out how accepting he is of these views by asking a further question:

> I don't know if you agree with your mother about this; tell me how right is she? How many marks out of ten would you give her?

This second question can be asked in relation to the mother's and father's responses but not others. It should not be asked before all of the attributes for each person have been given. Knowing that an accuracy score will be asked for is likely to change the response. This procedure sometimes shows how very restricted a child's view of himself is. There is a relationship between the way we see ourselves and the way we see others and repetitive responses may indicate a restricted construct system. One child who responded to the WAY questioning with the same, 'He's helpful, he's considerate, he's thoughtful' sort of statements, could say very little about other people. When asked what was special about his friends the response was that they were patient. The child knew they were patient because they did not laugh at his stuttering. The impression gained was that the child had to be helpful and so on because of his stutter and that he could only construe others on the basis of how they responded to his speech. Undoubtedly this very restricted way of construing others was a maintaining factor in his stuttering.

Ravenette ends by saying that he has now abandoned this technique in preference to other methods. This is mentioned because it emphasises the importance of *developing* techniques for our particular clients. It also shows the benefits of committing ourselves to a theoretical framework since we can 'invent a questioning technique and work out the psychological and theoretical implications afterwards' (p7). During the course of using a procedure, if we stumble across a different sort of question that evokes an interesting answer we can contemplate this. This new question may present us with different alternatives and, in this way, we may also keep developing and refining our methods.

(iii) Repertory grids

This section aims to discuss, very briefly, a few of the issues relevant to grid completion with children.

■ **Elicitation of constructs:** The methods discussed above can be used to elicit constructs. Using triads of elements may be difficult for children, but pairs can be presented and similarities or differences sought. Sometimes a child may find it difficult to focus on people but relatively easy to talk about a hobby. For example, one child could discuss quite easily how he selected which computer game to buy, but had nothing to say about familiar adults or peers. The constructs used in computer game selection were then considered in relation to people and several were found to have a sufficiently wide range of convenience: *interesting—boring* could be applied to people, whereas *with sound effects—without sound effects* could not.

Photographs of familiar situations and people can be used to elicit constructs. In a study of a seven-year-old with a physical disability **Morris** (1987) elicited constructs through photographs taken in the child's school. The photographs were selected so that children were shown with and without obvious handicap and engaged in a wide variety of activities. The child could not communicate verbally but by repeated sortings of the pictures constructs were negotiated. She was able to validate or invalidate the constructs that Morris verbalised with forceful non-verbal messages.

There is some controversy surrounding the use of supplied constructs. However those who justify their use do so on the grounds that the individual will use their own construct in response to the provided verbal labels (**Jackson and Bannister**, 1985b). A mixture of elicited and carefully selected supplied constructs can be used.

- **Grid completion:** Once sufficient constructs have been elicited a grid can be completed, although a child may have difficulty in understanding and using a large rating scale. A primary-age child may need to have each construct presented separately for each element and may benefit from having the rating scale written out or drawn. For example:

| very happy | happy | not happy / not sad | sad | very sad |

It is unlikely that the rating points for all the constructs could be named as easily as the ones in this example but the idea can be represented so that it applies to all constructs. **Shewell** (1987) used buckets of varying fullness to help some teenagers with Down's syndrome complete grids. The written form was adequate for the seven-year-old girl in **Morris**'s (1987) study.

When analysing children's grid data we can ask similar questions to those we might ask of an adult's grid but remembering that children may not have such well-articulated systems. Their constructs may have a narrower range of convenience so that they are forced to use middle ratings more often than adults. **Jackson and Bannister** (1985b) use ranking, which is one way of avoiding this problem. They also suggest that no more than eight elements are used since greater numbers may cause confusion and random responses.

(iv) Self characterisation

Young children may find it difficult to talk or write about themselves and it may not be an appropriate task for children under nine years of age. There is no normative data for young children and so it may be difficult to know what to make of children's responses. Self characterisations from children of nine to thirteen years have been studied by **Jackson** (1985) who has developed a method for classifying children's statements. The relative numbers of statements that fall into the different categories appear to be a function of the children's level of development and their success in coping with life. As optimally functioning children develop so they provide evidence that they are good psychologists and can think of positive things so say about themselves. Also they make statements that relate cause and effect in psychological terms. In the table below we list the categories suggested by **Jackson** (1985).

Table 4.2 Self characterisation categories

1	Self-esteem	Claims of competence or moral virtue.
2	Non-psychological statements	Behavioural statements, activities, physical descriptions.
3	Psychological statements	Any reference to thinking, feeling or other construing.
4	Personal history and future	Past or possible future referred to in psychological terms.
5	Conflict	Contradictory assertions or pairs of themes.
6	Insight	Awareness of own shortcomings and resulting problems.
7	Views of others	Child refers to view of self that is taken by others.
8	Psychological cause and effect	May be implicit, things linked but not understood as causally related, or explicit.

When we analyse a self characterisation we can look for items that fall into these categories as well as looking for themes. While researching character sketches, **Jackson and Bannister** (1985b) found a need to alter Kelly's original wording;

> Tell me what sort of boy or girl *Sally Jones* is. If you like I will be your secretary and write down what you say. Tell me about yourself as if you were being described by an imaginary friend who knows you and likes you and above all understands you very well. This person would be able to say what your character is and everything about you. Perhaps you could begin with *Sally* is . . . and say something important about yourself. Try to fill this page.

A character sketch written by a child must be treated with as much care and respect as one written by an adult. It is not a procedure to be used routinely but rather something that we invite a child to do when we wish to understand them in their own terms and we feel reasonably confident that they can cope with the task. The ability to look at oneself in the way that a character sketch requires does not come early, neither is it a skill that is acquired at any particular age. The content of sketches does develop with age but we must guard against looking for 'norms' rather than attempting to understand the child's view.

The self characterisation that appears below is short for a boy who has just entered his teens:

> "......... is a quiet boy but he is clever and polite and he gets on with his work, plus he is active. He is very sensitive on what people say."

He wants us to know that he is not as he seems, that is, that his quietness is not a sign of stupidity. He might be telling us that if it were not for his stutter we would know that he is clever. Most adults indicate that he is polite, not in what he says, but what he does, thus giving the impression that he needs to appear polite so that people would think well of him and, it is hoped, not ask him to talk. So it is interesting that he mentions politeness. There is a clue about the way the boy feels and this occurs at the end. If we take this sentence to be an enlargement of the comment on being polite then maybe politeness ensures that people speak well of him. The sketch is very short and it is what is *not* said that perhaps is the most significant. He has so little to say and includes nothing of his past or future. His family and friends do not get a mention, neither do his interests or hopes.

If we consider the categories that Jackson suggests then there are examples of positive statements about self, though of a non-psychological nature. His history and future are not mentioned. His sensitivity is a psychological characteristic but not accompanied by either insight or cause and effect. Quietness possibly conflicts with cleverness and politeness. No views of others are included.

This boy had great difficulty in construing other people and the character sketch suggests he is no better at construing himself. If the character sketch does reflect how this child attempts to make sense of himself and others, then there seems little hope that his stuttering will improve until he can elaborate his construct system so that he can become better at anticipating events. This boy might benefit from exploring ways of construing self and others. Constructs could then be elicited and a grid completed. The procedure would be slow, but might help the boy develop a stronger sense of who he is and how he can make sense of others.

Conclusion

The procedures that have been discussed in this chapter are not just for initial exploration. Many of them can be used throughout therapy as the need for better understanding emerges. The questions that we seek an answer to need to be clarified before we can select appropriate procedures. When we can match procedure to both client and tentative hypothesis then the process of exploration becomes absorbing and enlightening.

CHAPTER 5
THE MANAGEMENT OF YOUNG CHILDREN WHO STUTTER

Working with parents

In the previous chapter we considered the controversy over the issue of whether it is the child or the parent who is the client. Similarly, we must decide where the emphasis lies in therapy with different members of the family.

When considering whom we should work with, we are wrestling with theoretical as well as practical issues. If we believe that children find the conscious control of behaviour difficult, and that a child's behaviour is better understood within the context of the family, then we shall be more open to the work of those therapists who aim for second order change. However, if we favour the view that children can control their behaviour and that parents can be taught how to provide a good communication environment that reinforces fluency, then work that focuses upon first order change will be more appealing. In this chapter we shall consider both of these possibilities, since there is insufficient hard evidence to justify either approach to the exclusion of the other. The discussions of parental reconstruing and brief therapy are concerned with second order change. The section entitled, *Direct work with young children* focuses upon first order change.

It is not possible to make rules about which children will benefit the most from one or the other approach. However we offer the following justification for aiming at second order rather than first order change:

■ Many of the children who stutter also speak fluently much of the time. This leads us to question the appropriateness of routinely training children in fluency skills.

■ Even children who stutter severely may be markedly more fluent for a period of time following an initial interview where the problem was discussed openly by both the child and the parents. In these instances the potential for fluency as a result of change in attitude is demonstrated.

■ All fluency techniques encourage a focus upon speaking and this may do little to help the child develop constructs that are useful for making social predictions. The child may begin to construe in terms of speed, soft onset and so on instead of stuttering and struggling but still the focus is upon speech and so the child is likely to remain self-absorbed in difficult situations.

■ First order change is usually difficult, requiring discipline, regular practice and careful monitoring. Relapse is common and clients often blame themselves for not trying hard enough. Such experiences of failure and guilt are not beneficial to the developing child and can lead to the conviction that their stutter is untreatable.

■ We believe that therapy should aim ideally to produce the desired change in the shortest possible time. In this way the problems of dependency, and of therapy becoming a maintaining factor, are reduced. This aim is much easier to achieve with younger clients, but we are committed to finding ways of producing lasting change without a huge investment in therapy time by clients of all ages. We were educated in the tradition of long-term therapy and we developed our clinical skills within the context of short-term, intensive therapy. It is disappointment with long-term results that leads us towards different models of intervention. We are struggling to find out what it is that we do with our clients that really makes a difference, that really changes the way they see things and hence, their behaviour.

■ If stuttering serves a function within the family then relapse after therapy that deals only with the symptom is likely.

■ Part of our justification in pursuing second order change in preference to first order change comes from examining our own clinical records. When people have changed their view of the problem of stuttering the changes that they then make seem more permanent. Young children become fluent and need no symptomatic treatment at all. Older children and some adults manage to get off the roundabout of technique–practice–failure–recrimination–more technique–practice–failure and so on. It is perhaps important to add that some people do return to technique work after making a change of the second order. What is interesting is the way that they approach a technique: it is no longer a way of stopping stuttering but much more a means to a better understanding and use of the speech mechanisms. The realisation that the techniques are only as reliable as the person who uses them presents the client with a challenge rather than a desperate struggle.

In our view, second order change represents a therapeutic ideal and, unfortunately, we do not have the skills or understanding to be able to effect such a change with all clients. There are also children who have other developmental problems that might influence the development of fluency. When a child who stutters has delayed language development, a phonological problem or some other language-based difficulty, then we would recommend that these problems are worked with in such a way as to facilitate fluency. The occurrence of stuttering should never be a reason for stopping work on expressive language skills although it may indicate a need to consolidate rather than present additional new material. However, even when the cause of stuttering would seem to be language-based, we must not forget that other factors may be contributing.

The organisation of this chapter reflects our belief that work with parents should always come first. Work with the child on speech production may also be necessary but should never be prescribed routinely. We urge therapists to hold back from direct work until they are sure it is appropriate. It is easy to fall into the trap of thinking that you must *do* something about the child's speaking and then waste time with the meaningless practice of fluency techniques that have nothing to do with the child's speaking outside the clinic. The majority of the adults who come for therapy have had months, if not years, of such work. We must consider the possibility that the solutions to the problem that were offered by the speech therapists were themselves effective in maintaining the problem.

Considerations in working with families

(a) Who do we work with?

We believe that some contact with all family members is necessary in order that the therapist can understand something of their relationships and interactions. However we would not insist that all members are present for therapy. There are times when one parent is highly motivated for change and determined to keep all appointments and to carry out all negotiated tasks. When the other parent is relatively unconcerned or would find attendance a problem, due to circumstances outside their control, insisting upon their attendance may establish the wrong sort of relationship. Having the whole family present near the start of treatment may be enough to begin the process of change. Therapists must always remember that their clients come from family groups. The communication skills of a young child cannot be considered in isolation from the context in which they are developing and using these skills.

(b) What are the goals of therapy?

It is important that therapist and client agree upon the goals of therapy. Neither should aim too high. Discussion about goals of therapy helps to clarify issues such as how the parents view the problem; why it is a problem to them; how they think change will occur; acceptable steps along the way and how they will know when the problem is resolved. This information will help the therapist devise a therapy plan that is respectful of the client's understanding of the problem.

(c) How long should sessions be?

We feel that at least an hour is required for sessions that involve psychological exploration or reconstruing. Half an hour rarely allows enough time for therapist and client to get to grips with the problem. When therapy is focused upon direct speech work the length of session will be determined by the nature of the material and the child's ability to concentrate.

(d) What will the content of therapy be?

It may not be possible to describe the exact form that therapy will take, but it is important that clients have some idea of what is expected of them and the format of sessions. If clients disagree with the approach to therapy it is unlikely that they will be co-operative. Such disagreement may make it necessary that the therapist initially respect the clients' view.

(e) How many therapists will be involved?

It is unfortunate that very few speech therapists are able to work with a colleague, even when they consider it necessary. The value of supervision is discussed in the final chapter and we urge therapists to consider their own needs as well as those of the client. Working with families places additional stress upon the therapist. It can be difficult to keep up with all that is going on in a room where three, four or more people are interacting. When a colleague is observing through a one-way mirror, she can help the therapist to clarify aims and hence structure therapy. We may need to turn to other colleagues, such as social workers or family therapists, to learn how to support each other while we develop new ways of working with families.

Now that we have considered some of the principles of working with families we can turn to the content of sessions. There are families where the major problem seems to lie in the way that the parents construe both stuttering and the child who does it. Typically, the child has good language development and periods of normal fluency. There are a variety of personal views about stuttering that have an influence and these will have been explored in the early stages of therapy. In the section below some of these views are discussed.

Changing the family's construing of stuttering and other aspects of the problem

It is important to remember that people construe things in the way that they do for a reason, and that change may threaten core construing. This means that we must always attempt to understand how the clients' current beliefs make sense within their view of their world, and so, credulous listening is an important therapeutic skill.

Further, we believe that the therapist should be prepared to learn from clients. At times it is necessary to abandon hypotheses, even some of those that we feel particularly pleased with. If we remain open to new evidence, the process of change and development should continue, and that is our main concern.

Some clients will change the way they construe stuttering with ease. It is almost as if they require the therapist to give them permission to view the problem differently and then they are free to continue the job of being good enough parents. For others it is more difficult and it may be necessary to work slowly with several of the areas outlined below.

Information about stuttering can provide the parents with an alternative view of the problem. This can make stuttering more predictable and less catastrophic, hence reducing parental anxiety. First we listen to the parents so that we can identify the additional information that will help them make sense of the problem. If we are sensitive to their view we should avoid giving information that is discouraging. For example, when a couple seem to believe that they have more than their fair share of bad luck, they are unlikely to be reassured by the knowledge that three out of four children outgrow stuttering. It would be consistent for them to believe that their child would be one of the unlucky ones. Second, we must also gauge how much information is helpful: too much is likely to increase anxiety, since it makes stuttering seem too complicated.

When parenting seems a problem it may take time to work out where change can occur. It may be necessary to start with whatever problem the family is most concerned with before tackling stuttering. Sometimes parents may be helped by some apparently simple task that enables them to feel more competent. As they begin to see themselves as more able parents, so stuttering becomes less of a problem. Parent groups that aim to improve communication and resourcefulness in dealing with everyday problems can also provide long-term support and friendship.

Whose problem is it? For some people, the need to protect their children from pain is of upmost importance. Good parenting and protecting are seen as one and the same. If a child stutters, these parents may feel responsible and also fearful that teasing and ridicule will ruin the child's life. When parents assume that what worries them also worries their children they may benefit from discussing different problems and who it is who 'owns' them. Perhaps a common problem that provides a good example is the child's untidy room. Often the mother feels that the untidy room is her responsibility; the child may be unconcerned. One possible solution is for the mother to ignore the state of the room, and eventually (it is hoped!) it will become bad enough to bother the child. When the child loses things in the chaos, tidying up will have a purpose. In this instance, when the mother gives up the problem, she allows the child to experience the consequences of behaviour. However, it must not be underestimated how difficult this sort of change is for some parents.

Consideration of who 'owns' the problem may be threatening, but if it can be done alongside the exploration and elaboration of 'good parenting', then parents can learn to be caring and responsible and yet allow the child sufficient freedom to grow and develop. When the child is encouraged to learn from personal experience feelings of independence and competence may also improve communication.

Many parents find it difficult to acknowledge that what they think is a problem does not worry their child. Like the family in **Laing**'s poem (1972, p5)

> There must be something the matter with him
> because he would not be acting as he does
>   unless there was
> therefore he is acting as he is
> because there is something the matter with him
>
> He does not think there is anything the matter with him
>   because one of the things that is
>   the matter with him
>   is that he does not think there is anything
>   the matter with him
>
> therefore
>
>   we have to help him realise that
>   the fact that he does not think there is anything
>   the matter with him
>   is one of the things that is
>   the matter with him

There are also times when parents do not realise the extent of a child's anxiety about speaking. They may not realise how severely the child stutters outside the home, and so have little idea of the problem from the child's point of view. When a child is relatively fluent at home but stutters severely in school, therapy needs to take account of the school and involve appropriate teachers.

Behaviour is an experiment: Some parents have been persuaded by the current fashion for educating their children early and may mistakenly believe that they have a duty to teach their child, at the expense of experiential learning. When children become used to an adult always guiding and directing activities, they can begin to feel at a loss when this attention is not available. The child may rely too heavily upon adults for validation because of not being sufficiently in charge of spontaneous experimentation. Alternatively, the child may become frustrated, because all too often experiments are cut short by adult interventions.

Viewing behaviour as an experiment requires a different approach than that proposed by other psychological models. For example, if we think of a child clinging to his mother in the clinic, it may be easy to talk about separation anxiety; or to blame the mother for being over-protective; or to view her attempts at encouragement as reinforcing the clinging behaviour. Consideration of the question that the child poses by behaving in this particular way is more difficult. In order to guess at the child's experiment we must, to an extent, understand the child's construction of the situation.

To do this we must try to see things as the child does, and this may involve us seeing ourselves in a rather unfavourable way.

There may be something about us that is the opposite to a quality that his mother has. The room that we work in may look and smell like somewhere that has unpleasant associations. We may have tried to get to know the child too quickly and the clinging is a way of holding on to certainty in the face of unpredictability. Whatever the child's construction of the situation, we know that construing will be through all the senses and likely to be expressed behaviourally rather than verbally.

Seeing things from the child's point of view has already been mentioned in relation to difficult situations and is equally relevant to more enjoyable experiences. We can spoil a child's fun by imposing an adult construction. We can also devalue a child's experience by subtle communication that the adult construction is somehow the 'true' one. Many of us can recall times when our view of reality was considered unreliable, unless supported by an adult. **Crowe** (1983) in a book with a Kellian title, *Play is a Feeling*, (that is, it is not what you do but the way you construe it!) provides some wonderful examples of the realities of childhood. The experiences described were all memorable. The adults who retell them are able to construe the situations as if they were still children. They are talking about those experiences that somehow stand still within us and enable us to get in touch with the child that we once were.

Haley (1976) describes a task that he believes increases the mother's sense of 'objectivity' about her child. It also involves the mother in subsuming parts of her child's construct system.

> . . . the mother may be asked to hide something where it will take the child no more than ten minutes and no less than five minutes to find. She must repeatedly attempt this task until she succeeds. The mother must think through just how her child thinks, and how he thinks differently from her, to succeed. (p62)

Haley stresses the importance of the mother realising the *differences*, as well as the similarities, between her way of thinking and her child's, which fits well with Kelly's notion of bipolar constructs. Both of the authors referred to in this sub-section have written books that are of value to Kellian therapists, even though neither seems aware of Kelly's work.

There are many ways of listening but perhaps people have not had cause to consider them. When a child has a communication problem he may require to be listened to with extra consideration. Parents may benefit from tasks that will encourage them to develop their skills as listeners. **Pinney** (1983) coined the phrase 'Creative Listening' to refer to that very rare form of listening which occurs when someone gives total attention to another. Usually the listener is giving some attention to their reply, or is attempting to interrupt or maybe is busy doing something else. When people are listening creatively there will be pauses between speakers, since time will be needed to reflect and consider before answering with an alternative point of view. **Pinney *et al.*** (1985) claim that 'children need regular periods of total, non-directive and non-judgemental attention', and that when this occurs they become more confident and demand less attention from adults at other times.

Some families with older children engage in constant competition for speaking time and they may all benefit from use of the 'conch technique' (**Pinney**, 1983).

It is agreed that a conch shell or other similar object pleasing to the eye and touch be placed on a table in the centre of the group. All present agree not to speak, gesture or grunt unless holding the object. Anyone can pick it up to speak, but it should be agreed that whoever is holding it should stick to one idea on one topic. When they have finished speaking they return the object to the table for anyone else to take. (p5)

Once people have overcome their initial embarrassment they start to listen more attentively, there are often pauses before the shell is picked up, which suggests that people are not busy planning their responses while only half listening to the speaker. If the person who stutters can listen without thinking about their speech and can then speak without fear of interruption they may find communication more enjoyable.

There are other forms of listening, used by therapists with clients, that can be helpful for parents. Reflective listening encourages the listener to attend to meanings: the listener reflects back what the speaker has said. This is done at intervals and the speaker is reassured that the content of what has been said is understood and accepted.

When a child is upset, too often the feelings are ignored or trivialised and the adult focuses upon distraction. During a therapy session we all try to minimise interruptions, ensure a reasonable level of physical comfort and check that our furniture arrangements do not emphasise the different status between client and therapist. All of these factors can be taken into account by parents when listening to their children.

Carefully phrased questions can also indicate listening in much the same way as reflective listening. When eliciting constructs one may offer an implicit pole in the form of a question and this can help the client to clarify his own meaning. For example, if someone is struggling for the opposite to *listens well*, we might ask, 'is it *ignores others*?' The client may reject this and then settle for *doesn't understand others*, which will show us that, for this client, listening is more to do with understanding than with hearing.

It is interesting for people to think about all the different sorts of listening that they engage in, and to consider how they feel when on the receiving end of these listening behaviours. A focus upon listening should improve family communication and has the added advantage of taking the focus away from speaking. Also, if people are concentrating on receiving the speakers' thoughts they should be less concerned with how these are presented. Children who know they are being listened to may still repeat words or parts of words, but are less likely to force and struggle to get them out.

Extending the perspective of first-time parents: To an extent, the way we construe events is influenced by how permanent or temporary we believe them to be. A severe cold may cause unpleasant physical symptoms, but we know they will not last. Children may not have this knowledge and for them the present is often also the future. Only gradually do they learn to distinguish between those experiences that pass quickly and those that are more long-term. Inevitably parents lack experience with their first-born child. They may have difficulty in knowing what is a passing phase and what is a permanent characteristic. We all hope that the pleasing aspects of our children will last and that those that displease or pain us will be of short duration. Often parents are so concerned about the negative things that they start to try to get rid of them, with the result that the behaviours become more entrenched. When parents are able to stand back from the current problem and place it in a longer perspective they are more likely to be able to think of solutions.

Encouraging people to develop ways of solving problems is much more likely to help them in the long term than rushing to experts when problems arise. Reflecting upon previous problems and their resolutions reminds parents of their resourcefulness. Often the things that we resolved spontaneously are those where second order change has occurred and this should not just be dismissed as 'the problem went away'. The parents might have changed in some important way so that the problem was perceived differently, and hence a solution was found: or perhaps the thing they dreaded actually happened and they discovered that they could cope. A hypothesis-making and -testing approach can help parents, children and therapists handle their problems more effectively.

What does the child do that we call stuttering? When we view stuttering as a behaviour we can describe it reasonably well. When we think about the implications that 'stuttering' has for a person and their future we are aware of great variation and uncertainty. Often parents' concern is not so much with the actual behaviour but rather more with what it all means. Does it mean they have failed as parents and that their child is destined to a life of misery and isolation? When parents can see what the child does as related to current development and events, then they may be able to support the child, in precisely the same way as they offer support at other times of difficulty. They can respond to the child's need rather than to their own anxiety. For example, if the child is upset and stutters when talking about it, the parents can give the child time, acknowledge the feelings that are being experienced and then manipulate the situation to maximise the child's chances of fluency. This might involve the parent stopping whatever they are doing, turning the radio down, picking the child up and then moving to a comfortable place where the child can begin to explain why they are so upset. The parent may need to provide cues to help the child organise thoughts, although it helps the child to retain the responsibility for the content. We would not recommend that the parent always stop what they are doing when the child demands it but only when they realise the child is in trouble.

The CPC cycle, described in *chapter three* provides the framework for reconstruction in any of the above areas. The circumspection phase can use ideas obtained in a variety of ways, for example:

- Brainstorming—all sorts of possible solutions are written down without ordering or editing. The ideas can be realistic or far-fetched, the aim is to loosen construing around the problem;
- Exploration of problem, discussion of possible solutions;
- Describing solutions that other clients have used;
- Through reading appropriate material;
- Group discussion;
- Asking friends and relatives how they would tackle a similar problem;
- Observation of other people;
- Observation of the therapist when modelling alternatives.

The pre-emption phase involves client and therapist in the discussion, and then selection, of viable alternatives. The therapist's task is to check that the selected alternatives lead to an experiment that is meaningful to the client. This is why we are not able to prescribe a particular course of action for a particular difficulty. The process of working through the CPC cycle is important in that it can offer strategies for dealing with future problems. The final phase of the cycle involves the client in experimentation. The design of the experiment is important and the objective needs to be clear. If an experiment aims to increase a parent's pleasure in their child, then it can be invalidated if the parent evaluates success on the basis of the child's fluency rather than of their own pleasure. Alternatively, the experiment could have been doomed because the therapist had failed to take account of the parent's need to be constantly monitoring the child's speech. A shared activity, involving little or no speaking, might have been better.

There are other ways of encouraging reconstruing. Indeed many of the activities described in *chapter two* and *chapter four* are likely to begin the process of change. There is one further approach to achieving second order change that we wish to introduce. We have chosen to include *Brief Therapy* because it is compatible with personal construct theory and has obvious relevance to the problem of stuttering. Although it is not a well-tried approach with speech therapy clients, brief therapy has been used for some time by family therapists.

Brief therapy

It is not possible here to describe the theory and practice of brief therapy in sufficient detail to ensure that the reader can adequately use the approach. However, since it relates so clearly to stuttering, we hope that we have included enough to stimulate further reading.

The focus of brief therapy is on the communication between people and how this creates and maintains a problem. **Procter and Walker** (1987) describe the way problems are created when the initial solution fails and instead of something different being tried, more and more energy is directed to trying to make this solution work. Then, as

> individuals understand themselves to be failing in resolving the difficulty, it tends to be perceived as more serious, and consequently alarming. Accordingly more and more effort is indicated. Given the apparent gravity of the situation, a narrowing tends to occur in that range of actions people will consider as potentially applicable solutions. This reduction in resourcefulness, which may be accompanied by the recruitment of other family members (or outsiders) to help may render the problem even more central in life, interrupting the natural unfolding of the individual and family life cycle. . . (p4)

What is especially interesting about stuttering is that parents and child may be attempting different sorts of solutions: the child may put more physical effort into speaking so that repetitions become blocks; one parent may suggest that the child slows down; the other may react with annoyance and impatience. The first two reactions suggest a belief that stuttering is a physical problem with physical remedies; the third person seems to view the cause as laziness or to think that perhaps the child stutters just to annoy others. The child may be receiving conflicting messages concerning how best to overcome the problem, one parent suggesting slowing down and the other's impatience indicating the need to speed up.

The aims of brief therapy are relatively simple and confined to understanding 'something of the mechanism whereby people become stuck with problems and how to go about getting them unstuck' (**Procter and Walker**, 1987, p5). This contrasts with therapies that aim to cure or educate: even increased understanding or insight are not required of the client, although often these follow spontaneously once the change in the circular patterns of behaviour has been achieved.

In brief therapy the client is not instructed to stop using the solutions that are maintaining the problem since this is unlikely to be successful.

Trying not to do something can lead to an increase in the behaviour because of increased awareness. This in turn can lead to guilt or to the client rejecting the therapist's advice and thereby becoming more entrenched in the problem-creating approach. Instead, the therapist accepts the clients' view of the problem and encourages them in their solutions.

If we relate this to a family with a stuttering child, the pattern of interaction may be as follows. The parents may believe that the child's problem lies with particular sounds and that the solution is to teach the child how to say these sounds more slowly and easily. The parents' view is accepted, and they might be asked to check their theory by keeping a record of the child's stuttering during the next week. Thus prescription of the symptom stops the parents from behaving in their usual way since the stuttering becomes a desired behaviour, and they are no longer required to try to stop its occurrence. If the child is old enough to be included, then encouragement to stutter helps the parents in their task. This means that the stuttering becomes more of a voluntary behaviour, in that the child stops trying *not* to do it. If the child wishes to oppose the therapist or parents then this also leads to less stuttering.

If we take another example: a young child's stuttering may mystify the parents who are at a loss to explain it. Their puzzlement over the child's behaviour is likely to be expressed behaviourally and therefore maintains the problem. Their confusion can be acknowledged and they can be asked to keep a diary of the child's stuttering to help the therapist to make sense of the problem when they next meet. Parents are similarly restrained from trying to do anything about the stuttering when we reframe it, for example, by suggesting that it is a result of the child's sudden increase in vocabulary. In this way the stuttering is almost something to be pleased about since it shows that the child's language skills are developing.

It is usual for there to be a marked reduction in the symptom following its prescription. However, the therapist must continue to prescribe the symptom for a while longer to ensure that the old solutions are not tried again. It is also important that the therapist does not take credit for the improvement, since progress may be lost if the family feel that they have been tricked into changing. The therapist remains surprised at the progress and predicts a relapse which helps the family combine forces against the therapist as they attempt to prove the prediction wrong. This helps to maintain the new behaviours. We find the brief therapy model fascinating on several counts:

- Firstly, it has obvious applicability to the problem of stuttering.

- Secondly, many of the successful things that we have done with parents in the past could be explained by this model. For example, reconstruing stuttering so that it is seen as an indication of a new stage of language development may stop the parents worrying and, more importantly, trying to do anything about it.

- Thirdly, parts of **Van Riper**'s (1973) approach that we have found particularly helpful could also be construed within this model, for example, voluntary stuttering and desensitisation work.

- Fourthly, some of the sudden improvements following initial interview can also be explained. Discussing stuttering in an open and accepting way can reduce the person's need to hide it. Added to this is the client's knowledge that the therapist wants to see and hear the stutter. It is common clinical knowledge that most people who stutter will be more fluent with speech therapists than with other strangers. All of these factors may reduce the stuttering in the short term but long-term improvement will only occur if the changes in thinking are sustained over a period of time.

We can illustrate this by citing a rather puzzling example: a child who stuttered severely was refusing to continue to see his local speech therapist. His extremely worried parents contacted one of the authors, via a mutual friend. Rather reluctantly, it was agreed that we should all meet with the aim of giving the parents a chance to air some of their concerns. Regular treatment was not possible for geographic reasons, and we were all aware that a single meeting can raise expectations and increase dissatisfaction with local services to no useful purpose. However, the meeting took place, and both of the parents and the child were able to discuss a lot of issues that were distressing them concerning the child's speech and his future. Throughout the very lengthy meeting the therapist maintained a Kellian stance, listening credulously to all that was said and offering alternative constructions when they seemed appropriate.

Subsequent letters and phone calls revealed that the child's increase in fluency that had occurred during the meeting continued for all of the summer holidays. This was surprising and at the time difficult to explain, as was his sudden and very marked deterioration at the beginning of the school term, when he also decided to return to his speech therapist. The speech therapist was doing some form of speech control with the boy and perhaps this is what encouraged him to attempt again those failed solutions that involved struggle and blocking. This may also have been inadvertently encouraged either by the boy's teacher or by the child's expectation that he would stutter on returning to school. If he anticipated difficulty then he might return to the old solutions in the hope of averting stuttering.

The story does not have a particularly happy ending: the child's stutter got so much worse that the family decided that intensive speech control was the answer. The child is more fluent now, but is having to 'work hard at his speech'. Maybe a second order change will occur as a result of feeling more in control. If not the child is likely to tire of the hard work and so resort to his own failed solutions.

■ Finally, we find much in the brief therapy model that is compatible with personal construct theory. Both are respectful of the client's beliefs and require the therapist to listen in a credulous manner if the suggested task is to be appropriate. Second order change is aimed for and the interrelationship between thinking and doing is recognised. People are viewed as creative and resourceful and the therapist's job is to help clients become unstuck so that they can continue to develop and grow.

Brief therapy, as the name implies, produces change more quickly than is usual with personal construct therapy, and the procedures for terminating therapy are made more explicit. The steps in therapy are clearly described and the approach is apparently simple. However, as **Procter and Walker** (1987, p6) point out, 'the model [brief therapy] is far simpler to conceptualise than to apply'. On the other hand, Kelly's discussion of therapy is long and his ideas are quite complicated and at times difficult to grasp.

There will be occasions when the child's symptom reflects a problem between the parents. This is not a contraindication for brief therapy. The model can still be used to free the child from the problem, but further work will be needed to assist the parents in their relationship. This raises questions about professional boundaries and we leave it to individual therapists to decide how best to use their resources and those of supporting services.

Personal construct therapy with children

Whatever form our therapy takes with children we are aware of the importance of the adults in the child's environment. When a child is perceived as having a 'problem' then we can be pretty confident that someone experiences invalidation when the child behaves in the 'problem' manner. Problems exist only when they are deemed undesirable and therefore, to understand them, we consider both the complainant and the person complained about. Whenever possible therapy with children comes after some work with the adults who are important to the child.

In *chapter three* we discussed the contribution of Jackson and Bannister to our understanding of the way children develop their construct systems. The child's ability to construe self and others may not develop adequately if stuttering stops the child playing a role in relation to others in a variety of social situations. Difficulty in construing others will become apparent when exploring the child's understanding of their world. Since there is an interaction between our understanding of ourselves and of others, we can focus either on the child or on the people they meet in order to elaborate the child's construing of self and others. Some ways of achieving this aim are given below.

(a) Elaborating construing of self and others

Life history book. This is something that can be done at home as well as in the clinic. Photographs, pictures and mementos can be incorporated into the scrap-book which may be written by the child, with or without the help of others. A family tree invites the child to consider himself in relation to the rest of the family. Recording dates of birth and other important family anniversaries encourages an older child to take responsibility for remembering to buy presents or to mark these dates in other ways. This provides opportunities for testing hypotheses about people, since arranging treats for others involves us in construing their constructions of the event. Similarities and differences between family members can be explored and this may help the child to develop a stronger sense of self. Consideration of what people might be doing in three years' time will encourage the child to think about the way psychological characteristics influence behaviour.

Learning how to get to know people. In certain situations a person who stutters may construe themselves almost to the exclusion of others. They are so preoccupied with their fear of stuttering and their attempts to avoid it that they have little attention left for the other people in the situation. Ways of finding out about others can be discussed, practised in enactment, tried out in carefully designed experiments, and then elaborated and evaluated in subsequent sessions. (See chapter 7(d) *The experimental approach to stuttering therapy*.) Teaching social skills does not necessarily lead to more useful construing of others and so we recommend that each of the stages discussed above is given equal importance. Most children who stutter are able to speak relatively fluently with their peers and these experiences of successful social interaction can be used when finding ways of dealing with problems. In this way we validate the child's constructions of others and encourage learning from experience.

Reconstruing painful events. When people are free to decide upon their own life milestones they do not necessarily select those that psychologists choose (**Salmon**, 1985b). People who stutter may find that some of their personal landmarks involve speaking. Not only may they be painful but they may also never have been shared. The child may struggle to understand these painful situations while retaining some sense of self-worth and in the process arrive at a construction that does not lead to a better anticipation of future events. Sharing and updating these sorts of experiences can free the client from some of the pain as well as prepare them for the future.

The 'who are you?' technique (WAY). This is described in *chapter four* as an exploratory procedure but can just as well be used to encourage a child to think from another person's point of view. The child can be asked for important things about other people and these can be compared and contrasted with what they imagine others think of them. Sometimes children imagine that others focus only upon their shortcomings. In contrast, they may focus upon the strengths of others. Experiments can be designed to test and, it is hoped, invalidate the child's hypothesis that people are more concerned with their child's weaknesses than with their strengths.

(b) Understanding problems and offering alternatives

Children of primary school age may find that the familiar mediums of drawing and story-telling facilitate their understanding. Sometimes the child selects the medium through which to communicate with the therapist. **Dalton** (1987b) describes how a seven-year-old boy used a jigsaw of carefully designed shapes to describe his social network. Through this drawing it was possible for the child to work out a way of dealing with his best friend's departure to another school.

Ravenette (unpublished paper) invites children to draw their families when he wishes to explore how they see themselves in this context. Another technique that he describes requires the therapist to draw a straight line that bends downwards at one end. The child is then asked to make this into a picture which includes the self and four people who are important to them. The 'portrait gallery' technique is described in *chapter four* and this can be used in combination with the above techniques to explore a child's construing and to point to alternatives. Ravenette uses story-telling as a way of offering a child an alternative. The story contains correct biographical detail and addresses those issues that arise in the exploratory phase. A positive aspect of the child is commented upon and related to the context where the problem arises. Finaally, the child in the story is given a different name to the child in therapy. In this way the child is offered a realistic alternative without being covertly instructed to accept it. It is not possible to do justice to Ravenette's therapeutic procedures in such a brief discussion and so we recommend thhat therapists who are interested in his work refer to the original papers.

Conclusion

Personal construct therapy with children presents the interested therapist with a challenge. Our understanding of how children develop a system of personal constructs with which to make sense of their world is still quite sketchy. Therefore it is difficult to identify the ways in which a child's stuttering may distort this development. However, if we formulate hypotheses about the effects of stuttering, we can test these and in this way develop our understanding and skills. In personal construct theory children and adults are not viewed as opposites. They have in common an innate desire to be good scientists and so many of the principles and ideas that are used in therapy with adults can be modified for use with children.

Working with teachers

The principles that lie behind our work with teachers are essentially the same as those identified throughout this book. There are a few points to consider if we wish to develop a co-operative relationship.

- Teachers may have their own theories about stuttering and when we know what they are we are more likely to be able to intervene effectively.
- A speech therapist's job might look like a soft option to many harassed teachers and they may resent our attempts to involve them in therapy.
- A teacher who has tried to help the child and failed may feel that their professional competence has been undermined. They may look to the speech therapist to be told what to do.
- The solutions that teachers have tried may be maintaining the problem within the school.
- We are more likely to be able to alter the teacher's behaviour in relation to the child by offering alternative constructions of the child's behaviour than by requesting the teacher to behave differently. In other words, second order change will probably be more effective than first. Most teachers have so many demands to cope with, from children, other staff and parents, that no matter how much they wish to help the child, they are likely to forget what they have been asked to do.
- Sometimes visiting schools and reassuring teachers that they are not making the stuttering worse is sufficient to lead them to a more positive construction of their relationship with the children.
- Providing appropriate information can help the teacher construe stuttering and hence reduce anxiety.

We believe that part of our job is to help and support teachers and that this is most easily achieved when there is mutual respect. We recognise how fortunate we are in being able to spend time alone with our clients and that any information gained in this time must be treated with confidentiality. We must think carefully about how we can best serve the interests of our client; sometimes we provide a bridge between the teacher and the child, at other times we enlist the teacher's help in very specific ways or perhaps we are just available at the end of the phone. Whatever we decide should take account of the teacher's construing of the child and the problem. For the sake of the child we avoid placing more stress upon the teacher since this will add to the problem rather than solve it.

In the next section we consider ways of working directly with the child's verbal skills. It is likely that, even when the child has a specific language-based difficulty, attempted solutions are playing a part in maintaining the stuttering. The way that other people understand the problem will have an influence. Therefore we recommend that some work of the sort outlined so far in this chapter precedes any direct work with the child. If the focus is directed away from disfluency then the parents are more likely to provide an environment that facilitates communication.

Direct work with young children

Direct work with young children may be indicated when the child:

- Continues to stutter even though environmental pressures have been reduced;
- Is reluctant to talk to adults outside the family at an age when it is becoming necessary, for example, when starting school;
- Has age-appropriate language skills but seems to have problems in using them, such as sentence planning difficulty, slow word retrieval;

- Stutters severely and comes from a family who are unable to participate in therapy;

- Has difficulty with a particular type of speaking or group of people, for example, is fluent at home but stutters while reading or talking to teachers in school; or

- Has a cluttering type of speaking problem.

It seems important that a balance is maintained between the two options open to therapists, which are no work on speech at all against only working on speaking behaviour. Direct work is appropriate when assessment of the child's communication skills and the stuttering behaviour have led to the conclusion that structured fluent speaking experience is necessary. This may be needed because of a language-based problem or because the child has begun to construe speaking as difficult. Alternatively, it may be feared that the disfluency is pervasive enough for it to become a part of the child's usual behaviour. The experience of speaking fluently and easily is needed to reverse the trend, so that fluency once more becomes the norm, with stuttering the exception.

If assessment of the child's language skills reveals specific difficulties then these can be worked on in the same sort of way as for a fluent child with a language problem. Similarly, if the child has a phonological problem, standard treatment techniques can be used. In both cases attention should be paid to the complexity of the tasks, ensuring that easy speaking is encouraged to increase fluency.

The activities given below can be modified so that children may practise particular sounds, grammatical constructions, vocabulary, or whatever else is needed, to remediate their additional communication problems. We must stress that a child with an expressive language problem may be at risk of developing stuttering and that it may be a serious mistake to stop working on expressive language if stuttering occurs. Stuttering may indicate that the child is experiencing a sort of overload and so consolidation of the work done so far may prove helpful. Many adults who stutter are not good at making conversation and recall having been slow to talk. Whether or not they had particular difficulty with mastering spoken language or whether the stuttering limited their experience is a matter for conjecture. However, providing a young child with appropriate experience of talking about a variety of topics in a range of situations with different people will help, whether the problem is essentially one of attitude or of inherent difficulty.

Working systematically from simple imitation through to spontaneous speaking can be justified in several ways. If the therapist takes a behavioural view, then she is shaping the child's behaviour towards the goal of fluent speech. If this is the rationale, then careful attention should be paid to the grading of steps, the feedback given for correct and incorrect responses, and to the reinforcement that fluency attracts, both in the clinic and at home. If the aim is to increase the child's experience of fluency and provide practice in a variety of speaking situations with varied content, then the child's responses can be used to indicate the next steps to be taken. If the therapist wishes to understand the different speaking situations from the child's point of view she will continue to generate hypotheses during therapy and the testing of these will help in therapy planning. Whatever the theoretical stance of the therapist we do know that young children generalise fluent speaking within the clinic to their lives outside with much greater ease than teenagers or adults. Their worlds are also relatively smaller and so it is much easier to provide real-life situations for them.

A personal construct therapist has an additional therapy aim that has important implications for the ways in which activities are presented and the child's progress commented upon. We have already discussed the notion that people who stutter develop a construct subsystem to do with talking in general, and stuttering in particular. So our aim with children is to encourage the development of a variety of ways of construing themselves, other people, and situations where communication occurs. If they have begun to evaluate themselves according to how they speak, then we need to emphasise other aspects of the interaction and in this way elaborate social contact. Praising the child for fluency does not do this, it just places the child on the desired end of the *stuttering—fluency* construct. Comments about content or feelings are therefore more likely to help the child learn from his fluent experiences. Put another way, we hope the children will construe their fluent speaking not just in terms of fluency, but in ways that will help them to make socially useful predictions in the future.

Whenever we work directly with a child we keep in mind the notion of the *child as scientist*. We encourage experimentation and the development of a hypothesis-making and -testing approach towards problems. We attempt to see things from the child's point of view and to avoid forestalling their experiments. These ideas guide us when selecting activities and structuring therapy.

The steps and activities that we suggest in the following sections are derived from our clinical experience and a variety of other sources (**Cooper and Cooper**, 1985; **Heinze and Johnson**, 1985; **Ryan and Van Kirk**, 1978; **Shine**, 1980; **Stocker and Gerstman**, 1983; **Van Riper**, 1973; **Williams**, 1971). It is not suggested that each activity is used, but that activities are selected according to the particular needs of the child. Fluency is the aim and so careful attention must be paid to the demands that each task makes of the child. Big jumps in level of difficulty are to be avoided. It is up to the therapist to decide when to move on to another type of activity and also whether or not she wishes to use some sort of tangible reward.

There is agreement that speech should be modified as little as possible to achieve easy, fluent speaking. Most approaches use a combination of modelling and systematic control of the complexity of utterance to facilitate easy, relaxed speaking. **Gregory** (1986, p349) recommends 'slower rate with easy initiations and smooth movements', supplementing these techniques with breathy onset when necessary. **Cooper and Cooper** (1985) suggest using whatever Fluency Initiating Gestures (FIGs) the child finds helpful. **Ryan and Van Kirk** (1978) reinforce fluent speech while gradually increasing the length and complexity of utterances.

The procedures following disfluency do vary: **Costello** (1983) provides feedback by verbal means, such as 'stop' or by the removal of tokens: the child is not given an explanation since this seems to lead to confusion and most children quickly understand the behavioural response. In Ryan and Van Kirk's programme the child must begin again at the same step. **Heinze and Johnson** (1985) suggest that stuttering indicates that the child is having difficulty and consolidation should follow. Whatever the clinician decides it is important to be consistent and to focus on the things that the child is doing right and not on the mistakes that are made. **Williams** (1971) emphasises the importance of not focusing upon the speaking behaviour, but rather on the underlying cause of difficulty. So, for example in the later stages of therapy, if the child stutters when retelling an event the therapist should comment upon the feelings that interfered with fluency: 'You're still feeling upset about hurting yourself' or 'It made you feel very cross', rather than commenting on speaking.

Therapy

We suggest that any activity to be done at home is modelled first by the therapist. Then the parent should try the activity with the therapist watching. If the parent has obviously understood the object of the task and is able to do it in an appropriate way then no further instruction is needed. If the parent changes the task so that, for example, a finger game becomes a test of the child's knowledge of the rhyme then further demonstration by the therapist is needed. It is not desirable to criticise the parent but rather to comment on the things that were done correctly and demonstrate the difficult part again. For example, 'You spoke very easily and slowly during that rhyme and your child obviously enjoyed listening to you. Would you watch me again while I show you the sort of thing that you can say to encourage him to join in'.

It is very important that parents see therapists as supporting them and not as criticising them. The skills that they have should be recognised and used and we must have the humility to learn from them as well as to teach.

First stage: familiar material in unison

- Familar children's songs
- Nursery rhymes
- Finger and action rhymes

There is no shortage of materials for these activities: there are numerous rhyme and song books that are easily available. It may help children if the parents bring in favourite rhyme books to use at this stage.

Homework: Parents can continue with the same activity once a day and at any other times when the child becomes particularly disfluent. The physical closeness that occurs when sharing the same book, or doing the same actions, and the simplicity of the task should develop their relationship and, it is hoped, ensure a quick return to greater fluency.

Second stage: imitation

In this stage the child starts by imitating single words and builds up to a short story.

Single words: There are different ways of making this activity interesting, for example, rolling a car or ball to the child and saying the word with the child imitating the word while returning the object. Using a bag in which to place small objects that are named as they are pulled out, or placing a number of picture-cards face down and letting the child choose which ones to turn over, are other ways of achieving this objective.

There is an ever-increasing supply of pictures to use in therapy and those that the child can keep are perhaps most useful at this stage. Good examples of pictures to photocopy are the two *Pictures Please* books (available from Winslow Press).

Short phrases and sentences: The same pictures or objects can be used to increase the length of the utterance; for example: 'car, a blue car, it's a big blue car, I would like a blue car like that'. The activity can be varied by using materials like Fuzzy Felt, Lotto, What Goes With What Lotto and so on. At this stage it is *not* recommended that they are played as a competitive game.

Pictures depicting everyday events can also be used. **Heinze and Johnson** (1985) differentiate between pictures with an emotional content and those without, and recommend using the latter first. For example, a child with a hurt knee would constitute an emotional picture, whereas a tree growing in the garden of a house would not.

Retelling a story: The child repeats what the therapist says about a sequence of pictures, taking one picture at a time. It is important to keep the pictures simple and not to use too many to make up the sequence. Probably three or four pictures is enough, with no more than two short sentences for each one.

Homework: Children may not wish to play such structured games with their parents and when this is the case it is a mistake to try and make them do so. When either or both parents have observed the therapy sessions they will understand the aims. Different activities can be discussed or tried out with the therapist watching, until some suitable ones are discovered. For example, objects from around the house can be put in a bag or special box during the day, then these can be named and talked about; for example: 'a toothbrush, David's toothbrush, David's red toothbrush, David's toothbrush lives in the bathroom', and so on. At this stage the emphasis is upon fluent speaking experience and going over familiar material is inevitable. Most children do not mind imitating and parents should refrain from rushing on to spontaneous speaking, even though the child may be completely fluent when imitating.

Third stage: stereotyped sentences

The intermediate stage between imitation and spontaneous speaking is highly predictable speaking with just one or two chosen words. Much of the speaking that accompanies picture and board games is of this type; for example, 'I've got a car, do you need a car? Oh look, there it is', and so on. If children are asked to use the same sentence forms as the therapist then they will practise saying sentences without having to generate them. Some of the activities may be competitive. **Heinze and Johnson** (1985) suggest that the therapist ensures that the child wins, while demonstrating how to lose with grace. They recommend keeping comments about winning to a minimum and then when the child wins saying, 'Oh! You won and I lost. Oh well, I had fun anyway. It's fun to play even if you don't win. Maybe I'll win next time, (p13). The therapist is also instructed to make the occasional mistake; for example, 'I found a pig. Oh! I mean a goat'. This gentle introduction to the acceptability of mistakes and losing aims to reduce high self expectations when they are a problem, and to increase tolerance of frustrating experiences.

Fourth stage: spontaneous speech

Once the child is able to produce stereotyped sentence forms with one or two words of his own then gradually the amount of spontaneous speech can be increased. The same materials can be used but the therapist varies what she says so that the child no longer follows her lead. As the games become more spontaneous so the amount of speaking can gradually increase. Short stories can be generated from sequence pictures and everyday scenes and then questions and answers or descriptions can be extended to encourage the child to generate short utterances. For example, the child can describe what he can feel when fingering an object hidden in a small material bag. Asking questions to find out which of six animal pictures they are thinking of can be done with quite young children, for example, 'Is it furry? Has it got big eyes?' Similarly pictures of different people, sorts of food and furniture can be used.

Association Lotto can be turned into a descriptive game when the small card is described and its partner thus identified; for example, 'I've got something that's brown, has four legs, is very big'. Guessing can be discouraged until two, then three and then four things have been said about the object.

Summary

The suggested levels of difficulty to work through are:

- single words
- two words
- short phrases
- short sentences
- connected short sentences (either sequence or description)
- questions and answers

In addition attention should be paid to the nature of the content. The child is more likely to become involved and excited when the material has personal significance and this may lead to disfluency. Therefore initially the sequence should be worked through with unemotional material and then the latter items tackled again with more significant content. Pictures of the family and questions about the family and child should come later. Gradually the child is encouraged to take more verbal responsibility.

It is a good idea to start to reduce the predictability once the child has worked through each stage in a structured manner. To increase the complexity of the situation, it is useful to include cards that are not needed for the game, to increase the number of mistakes that you make, or occasionally drop cards or get in a muddle. If fluency breaks down during these activities try to find out what it was that stressed the child; this requires looking for patterns, testing hypotheses and then providing more practice at whatever is proving a problem. Whenever the child starts to stutter, consolidation at an earlier stage may be required.

Suggested activities and games

- Picture Lotto
- Association Lotto
- Happy Families
- Pairs
- Simple number games
- Picture and number dominoes
- Jigsaw puzzles can also be used when pieces are placed upside down and then named or described when turned over
- Guess Who (MB Games, Milton Bradley Ltd, Gwent.)

Homework: Suitable games that the child has at home can be played with the same careful restraints on the amount of spontaneous language used. It may work better for the parents to extend the basic idea of simple stereotyped sentences to activities around the home; for example, setting the table, tidying a room or getting dressed could all be done with a very simple running commentary that the child could join in with. If this sort of activity provides a good context for fluent, stereotyped utterances something more ambitious could be tried, for example, the discussion before, during and after a shopping trip. A big expedition should be left to a later stage since the noise and other people would provide too much distraction. However a trip to the local shops to buy just a few items could work well. Firstly, a shopping list can be written: 'I think we need a bag of sugar, what do you think we need?' with each person taking a turn to suggest one item. Then, while shopping, mother and child can take turns to direct each other, for example, 'You get the butter', 'Here's the sugar'. Once home, the same sort of things can be done while putting the shopping away. This type of activity can lead easily into questions and answers when the child is ready for more demanding speaking. Collecting items during the day, for looking at in the evening, can be extended to encourage very simple utterances.

Fifth stage: learning to cope with communicative pressure

This stage consolidates the fluency experienced in the previous stages while gradually increasing the amount of distraction and potential pressure. **Van Riper** (1973) talks about the need to toughen the child up so that he can retain fluency even when experiencing 'fluency disruptors'. We are all aware of how much easier it can be to talk to a familiar adult in a familiar situation than to talk when there are a variety of competing demands. A great deal of children's talking occurs in far from ideal situations. For example, there are often height differences, other equally determined speakers, strong rushes of emotion and all the while the child is using far less practised skills than the adult.

The suggestions that follow are intended as guidelines. Each therapist will be able to include other activities that are particularly relevant to her clients. **Heinze and Johnson** (1985) refer to this stage of therapy as 'desensitization'. The child is taken through the steps of imitation to formulation with each type of additional distraction. If the child has difficulty in speaking fluently when distractions are introduced, it would seem appropriate to follow Heinze and Johnson's suggestions. However, if the child does not seem sensitive to some distractions then these need not be worked on so extensively. When a child is disrupted it is helpful to consider which aspects of the situation are causing difficulty. These can then be incorporated into other variations. For example, a child may begin to stutter when the therapist applies some time pressure. It may be the time pressure or the way of speaking that bothers the child. Experimentation should determine which it is and then further experience can be given and the child helped to develop strategies for coping. The therapist might say, 'When I have to clear up quickly I do one thing at a time; what shall we start with?' or 'When people talk to me very quickly I try to talk extra slowly. Can you talk slowly while I talk quickly?'

It is worth considering **Shine's** (1980) approach towards the generalisation of clinical fluency. He uses a 'surprise box' of little objects at the end of each session so that the child speaks spontaneously. The fluency experienced in the preceding part of the session will often carry over into this activity and so the child has the experience of formulating fluent utterances early on in therapy. **Costello** (1983) describes the 'within session generalization probe' which is a three- to five-minute period within every second to third session. The therapist describes it as 'taking a break' and all treatment contingencies are withdrawn. The child and therapist engage in conversation and the therapist covertly records the child's disfluencies and in this way the child's ability to maintain fluency is examined. Obviously it is not possible to tell how extensive generalisation is but at least some impression is gained as to 'whether the improved fluency observed during treatment is beginning to show durability, at least within the treatment environment' (p93).

Another advantage of introducing some spontaneity early on in therapy is that the therapist can observe the strategies that the child is developing to deal with fluency disruptors. Children have been observed to slow down their rate of speech when attempting novel grammatical structures. Articulation rate may be slowed when tackling a polysyllabic word. The child may use non-verbal means to indicate their desire to speak, or repeat a word, rather than a syllable when formulating an utterance. Observation of these sorts of strategies is encouraging and may indicate that therapy can proceed in somewhat larger steps than currently used.

Distractions, pressures and activities

The activities used in former stages can be used again with the same regard for the gradual increase in the demands made of the child. We hope that less time will be required at each level, so that a short amount of imitation followed by single words is quickly followed by phrases and sentences. The child should be able to formulate questions and answers and generate 'stories' as final steps with each type of distraction.

Addition of people.   People can be invited to attend the therapy sessions, initially to observe and then to join in. The best order might be: family members; familiar adults; unfamiliar adults; familiar peers and unfamiliar peers. It can be advantageous to invite other disfluent children and their families who are at a similar stage in therapy or who are being seen for review. Both families will benefit from the contact and if time is set aside to talk with the two groups of parents some helpful exchanges might take place.

Competing noise.   Initially competing non-verbal noise can be introduced, for example, pencil tapping, typing in the background, or music. Once the child is able to maintain fluency with these noises verbal distractions can be introduced. It is important to remember that we find it much more difficult to shut out spoken language than any other noises and that it becomes increasingly difficult as the material becomes more relevant to us. For example, it is much easier for a child to cut out the voice of an unfamiliar adult who is talking about obviously adult topics than to ignore a familiar voice talking of things that interest the child. The best example that we are all familiar with is the sound of our own name. The sorts of verbal distractions that could be used are radio, songs, nursery rhymes and, if possible, television with first adults' and then children's programmes. Finally, the accompanying parent could hold a conversation with someone in the room while therapy continues.

Playing and talking.   The children's focus of attention is shifted away from the speaking activities and onto physical activities that they enjoy. These can be table-top activities, such as drawing, colouring, cutting, playdough, jigsaw puzzles and so on, or more energetic, depending upon the child's interests and needs. Playing with a ball, cars, bricks, sand or water may be more appropriate to the children's interests but may fail to stimulate conversation.

Interruptions and surprises.   Many adults who stutter cannot cope with the unexpected and to make things worse they often have rather narrow expectations of others and so are quite frequently confronted by things they had not predicted. As the person who stutters becomes more experienced at stuttering he often develops very strong convictions about the sorts of things he can and cannot do. He may cope with the uncertainty that stuttering brings to his life by constructing rigid rules about how he and others will behave and when people or events fail to conform he is at a loss to know how to proceed. Providing the child with opportunities to experience a variety of interruptions and distractions and to learn that they can cope with them without anxiety and stuttering is important, not only for fluency, but also for developing a tolerance of uncertainty.

Although children need to have their predictions about important people and events validated they do not benefit from things always being exactly as expected. The therapist is not going to suddenly behave in a manner contradictory to her usual manner, but she may add a few distractions, for example: dropping pencils; moving around the room; talking with her back to the child; turning away while he is speaking and so on. One verbal five-year-old, with an extremely attentive mother, found it very difficult to speak fluently with his teacher when other children were also clamouring for her attention. He was an only child who was used to having full listener attention when he spoke. He benefited from the experience of maintaining fluency with varying degrees of listener interest but also needed to be able to express his anger at not being the centre of attention. His teacher helped him by giving a clearer message about who she was talking to and by making all the children wait their turn and not compete with each other for her attention.

The interruptions can be organised with other colleagues so that people knock on the door, phone during the session, interrupt to ask questions and so on. When the child has shown that he can cope with all these different interruptions the therapist can interrupt him, ask him to repeat, ask for clarification, pretend not to understand and so on.

Contradictions. Can also be introduced by the therapist making deliberate mistakes in what she says or what she does. The child can be questioned and disagreed with.

Time pressures. The feeling that you must speed up is one to which people who stutter are very sensitive and which they invariably find extremely disruptive. At home time pressures are often difficult to avoid since different children make different demands of their parents, who may be struggling to keep to some externally imposed timetable. Time pressures are also a feature of school life and children impose them upon themselves when they compete to do things the fastest or communicate impatience when kept waiting. In therapy the child can be given instructions to do things with a time limit and also given experience in dealing with less obvious time pressures:

- The therapist can increase the rate of her own speech, look at her watch while the child is talking, look impatient;
- Verbal instruction to hurry up, such as, 'Hurry, we've still got lots to do';
- Being busy tidying up while the child is talking;
- Using a stop-watch to check that a child says an agreed number of words in a set time. This could be picture naming and then specific requests, for example, all the children you know, the things you could find in a food/vegetable/toy shop and so on. The number of words can be increased one at a time if the child is fluent. The child can also compete against himself by seeing how many words he can say in a specified time, or compete with the therapist.

It is important to work through these activities systematically so that the child remains fluent and begins to learn how fast he can go and withstand the pressure of time.

Increasing the relevance of the content. Much of the work so far has used pictures and games that do not have any emotional significance for the child. It is generally true that children are more disfluent when excited or under some sort of emotional stress. The parents should be able to help the therapist select content of some emotional significance to the child. For example, if the child has recently hurt himself pictures of a child going to the doctor could be used; if the child has moved house, lost something, or had a day out somewhere, then these experiences can be discussed. The child's feelings can also be elicited: 'That must have made you feel sad; what else makes you feel sad?' **Shirley Hughes** (1979, 1981, 1984) has written several beautifully illustrated books that tell stories around important events in children's lives. Puppets or miniature people may be used to encourage construing of others as well as allowing the child to distance himself a little from the emotion under discussion.

Competition. For those children who need to win it may be important that they learn to lose. **Heinze and Johnson** (1985) suggest three stages: (1) bringing the child close to losing; (2) introducing verbal competition while the child is still winning, and (3) contriving that the child finally loses. They recommend that the child should still win more often than lose and that he should finish the session with a win. Once the child can tolerate losing without stuttering then the parents can begin to win occasionally when playing games at home.

Change of location. This is an important variable since it is likely that the child has learnt to associate the clinic room with easy and relaxed speaking. Maintaining the easy speaking within a variety of situations is an essential prerequisite for fluent speaking in real-life situations. The sorts of changes in location that might be appropriate are: keeping the door open; a different room; working in the corridor; using the clinic play/waiting area. Finally these different locations can be used while different disruptors are introduced, such as time pressure, distractions and so on.

If the child is sensitive to any other disruptors these can be worked on in the same manner, the therapist remembering always to leave questions and answers and formulation of connected sentences until last. Many young children will not need to work in such detail since they will spontaneously generalise the fluency experienced in the clinic to situations outside. As a general rule the older the child and the more severe the stuttering, the more time needs to be spent on very carefully working through the whole range of speaking situations.

This stage of therapy may be adapted to groups of school-age children. Many of the disruptors will arise spontaneously and so care must be taken to structure the tasks, otherwise the therapist may lose control of all the variables that have an effect upon fluency.

Sixth stage: transfer of fluency to real-life situations

So far the therapist has used pictures and games to stimulate verbal expression while setting very definite limits upon the form and content. The child now needs experience in talking more spontaneously in a wider variety of situations. The materials used in the clinic can be extended to include stimuli that the child will find more interesting or amusing. Examples of pictorial materials that may encourage more spontaneity are given below.

LDA
What's Wrong Cards
Why—Because Cards

What Would You Do?
See How You Feel

Winslow Press
Advanced Sequences
Family
Topic Bank
School

See also two reference books: *All The Games Kids Like* and *Clinician's Choice*. *Pictures Please!* are two books with pictures to photocopy; one is for language and the other for articulation work, but both can be used in a variety of ways. All of these are available from Winslow Press.

Creata (via Winslow Press)

Fred's Family
Patch Pictures
Unusual Angle Photographs

DLM
Open Sequence Cards
Reaction Cards
Shape Recognition—Plastic Shapes

Materials available from toy shops
Fuzzy Felt
Vinyl reusable pictures
Board games involving discussion

Equipment of the sort listed can be used to encourage longer utterances with more abstract content. Questions can be asked where the child will have to generate his own answers rather than just one of the stereotyped responses that he used earlier. The materials can also be used to generate questions of a more personal nature, such as 'This boy looks sad, what makes you sad?' or 'what makes mummy sad?' and so on. Some of the distractions used in the last stage can be incorporated when the child can maintain fluency with these more varied activities.

Standard clinic equipment can be used. Dolls, tea sets, doll's house, playmat, cars, 'Playpeople' and so on can all be used to provide the context for more spontaneous conversation.

The activities should not be too absorbing since this may reduce the child's inclination to talk, neither should they encourage solitary play. When the child engages in play with either the therapist or the parent it is hoped that conversation will arise. Many children enjoy walking with an adult and talk much more than they would when playing. Other children may talk more when engaged in a 'real' task and so washing everyone's coffee cups or tidying the toy cupboard may be a better activity. If there are facilities for simple experiments with water or other materials these can be used at this stage. Real experiments encourage running commentaries and propositional speaking. The Usborne Publishing Company, London, produce some books that describe simple experiments with everyday objects and materials. As before, when the child is able to speak fluently and easily distractions and disruptions can be introduced.

The next step aims to provide experience in some of the situations that people who stutter often find difficult and that can be stressful for the young child in school. The amount of formal speaking required of children at school will vary within each class and from one school to another. A visit to the child's school should help identify where particular difficulties lie. Some ideas for therapy are given below.

■ Retelling familiar stories with the aid of pictures. (First check which stories the child is familiar with and hears at home.)

■ Enactment of situations and events that occur in the child's daily life. Easy situations should be tackled first and then difficult ones. With older, school-age children a definite hierarchy can be made and worked through. Roles can be exchanged so that the child sees the therapist model alternative ways of behaving in the situation and hears her use an easy speaking pattern. Exchanging roles also gives the child an opportunity to see things from another point of view which may help to make the situation more predictable. When possible use props to make the situation more realistic. Encouraging the child to set the scene in some detail also provides practice at describing people and situations.

The retelling of events in the child's life is often required in school. They may be asked to tell a group or class of children their 'news', or to describe an experience or event. The child can be encouraged to bring things to the clinic to talk about. Parents can keep the therapist informed of any events that interested the child. Events that were in some way difficult for the child should not be attempted until he can speak easily about those that were pleasurable.

If the child has difficulty talking in any of these situations they can be acted out either in role play or with puppets and the child can experiment with different ways of handling the situation. For example, if the child cut his knee and stuttered when telling his mother what happened, this can be acted out with the child taking the mother's role and then later being himself. The therapist can model easy speaking while she takes the child's role. If the mother finds these sorts of situations difficult, she can take part as well. Sometimes re-enacting a stressful situation attaches a significance to it that may be counter-productive. If this is the case a similar sort of situation could be acted out with puppets and once more roles could be exchanged. What is important is that the child sees and hears a relaxed and easy way of speaking and that alternative ways of dealing with the situation are presented. The mother may benefit from seeing these alternatives and, we hope, should develop strategies for dealing with these sorts of situations. It may be that taking her upset child upon her knee is more important for fluency than any amount of carefully worded questions. She may feel that it is wrong to ask the child to wait before talking and will find it helpful if the therapist models this; for example, 'Oh! you are upset. Come and sit on my knee and then tell me what happened'. This does not in any way criticise the child or focus on the difficulty with speaking but does allow a few seconds to organise thoughts as well as providing the necessary physical reassurance. Disruptors can be introduced at an appropriate time.

So far, transfer has focused upon extending the child's use of language within the clinic and it should now be possible to prepare for fluent speaking outside. Many children will have spontaneously generalised their clinical fluency and will only need to work on one or two problem areas. However the school-age child with severe stuttering may well need to continue to work within a careful structure in order to become more fluent in all speaking situations.

There may be specific problems at school or playgroup and these must be investigated by the therapist. Sometimes people unintentionally put press-ure on the child by trying to help him out and speak for him. Many adults can recall the fear of having to speak before the class. A teacher who knows of this fear may have decided not to ask the child to speak in this context but has never discussed it with the child. This means he continues to live in fear of being asked and never has the chance to discover that he can stutter a bit and that it does not matter. Helping teachers and playleaders gain sufficient understanding of stuttering so that they can avoid needless pressure is important. Talking freely about the problem with the child and teacher can help them negotiate the best ways of handling difficulties when they arise.

The therapist can also help by providing a bridge for the child between the clinic and school. Structured work on ever-increasing demands, such as content, audience size, amount of competition, can help the child generalise what he has learnt in clinic to the school. Fortunately most children of primary school age enjoy having a visitor in school and the other children delight in being allowed to participate in games and activities that the therapist organises. Very rarely is the child victimised for needing special help: more usually it seems to increase the child's status. Many of the children with whom we have worked have only required a couple of visits in school. This has been sufficient to provide the teacher with a practical understanding of the child's problem and for the child to generalise his fluent, easy speaking. It is interesting that some children have been helped more by playing host to the therapist and introducing her to his life at school than by systematic practice.

One child in particular who springs to mind took a great delight in showing the therapist around the school and classroom. In the process he was required to introduce her to teachers and children. The therapist manipulated the visit so that the child had practice at reading, description, story-telling, game playing and introductions, as well as a short discussion at the start to determine how disfluencies were to be managed. The child spoke fluently throughout the visit and continued to do so with only very minor returns to disfluency. During a subsequent telephone conversation with the teacher the management of the remaining part of the problem was discussed. It must be added that the child's mother gained a good grasp of the child's communication problem and that she modified her behaviour quite considerably to the benefit of his speaking. What was important was that she was able to provide an excellent link between home, clinic and school, and she helped the teacher as well as the therapist.

The importance of providing a bridge between the clinic and the outside world must not be underestimated. Relapse after therapy is inevitable if attention is not paid to thorough transfer. Kelly stresses the importance of not merely cataloguing events but of understanding what they mean to the individual. In just the same way transfer is not a case of merely working through a list of activities but is concerned with helping the individual see similarities between different people and events so that he can make socially useful predictions.

Often parents are very good at showing children these similarities. If one listens to a mother introducing her child to a new situation then often she refers to those things that are familiar first: 'Oh look, they've got a car/doll/ball, just like ours'. This is more usual than 'Here's a toy you've never seen before'. The second utterance may well come after some common ground has been established and the mother now feels that direction towards something of novelty value is appropriate.

When a mother has been involved in therapy and has understood the aims as well as how these translate into behaviour she is often the best person to provide a bridge between the clinic and playgroup. Many playgroups foster parental involvement and the playleaders are often receptive to the parent's contributions. When the mother can be involved in transfer by providing bridges for the child she not only saves the therapist a great deal of time but she also develops the skills necessary to help her child cope with many of the new situations that arise as he develops greater independence. This is an important factor when long-term objectives are considered.

In some schools parents are encouraged to help in the classroom and at lunch times. When this is the case parents can help with transfer within school. Even when parents are not encouraged to participate in the child's education there are still opportunities for meeting the teacher and ways of implementing transfer can be discussed.

The amount of speaking that children do outside the home and school varies considerably with age and life-style and this must be taken into account when planning the next stages of therapy. Puppets and role play can be used to explore different ways of behaving and to give practice before the 'real' event. The strategies that obviously help the child should be identified and then practised so that they become a part of his usual repertoire of behaviour. Those strategies that are part of the stuttering problem need replacing; for example, if the child rushes when asking for something in a shop then he needs practice at planning and taking his time. If he would run up to *anyone* to ask for directions he must learn to look and make judgements about who might be a receptive person. Encouraging a focus upon content, the listener and dimensions of speaking other than fluency are all important aspects of any transfer activity.

Seventh stage: continuing the process of change

The issues involved in maintaining change and in continuing to develop vary with the age of the child. Young children usually become fluent after very little therapy; however we recommend that contact is maintained for a couple of years. In this way we remain available, if needed, and also we are able to evaluate the long-term effects of our therapy. Telephone calls every few months may be all that is needed.

When therapy has been essentially successful only small problems are likely to be presented at follow-up sessions. If the ability to solve problems has been developed during therapy then usually parent and therapist can work out solutions to the current difficulties and with time these problems diminish.

Sometimes the therapist may feel that the parents would benefit from further support and help in more successful parenting. Some health clinics run parent groups and there are some privately organised groups. For example, The Parent Network in London are setting up groups on a local basis; The Adlerian Society (also in London) has a contact list of leaders who run parent study groups; some speech therapists may consider running their own groups for parents of children with communication problems.

There are a variety of possible patterns of relapse. The child may be fluent for a while and then start stuttering again for no apparent reason. Alternatively, stuttering may have started to increase gradually as soon as regular contact was stopped; or the child remained fluent and then started to stutter again when the family moved or the child changed school. A hypothesis-making and -testing approach seems more appropriate than merely recycling the child through previous stages.

The child may be stuttering again because he has gone back to evaluating himself and others on the basis of speaking. This may have been triggered by an apparently minor event and therefore does not necessarily indicate a need for further direct work. A session with the parents and child may indicate that previously failed solutions are being attempted and instructions to monitor or encourage the stuttering is all that is needed (see section on brief therapy). In this instance, therapy that focuses upon speaking might maintain the problem. When the therapist holds the view that behaviour is purposeful, that it asks a question and that it can be understood by careful exploration of the family construct system and the child's construing, then a solution should be found. We maintain that it is impossible for a therapist working on her own to solve the problems presented by the client with severe and persistent stuttering. In these cases it is often helpful to enlist the aid of either a psychologist or a family therapist.

whom we cannot help. Whatever we do, they continue to stutter as much as before. It is not helpful to keep referring someone from one agency to the next and if after careful consideration the conclusion is reached that, at present, there is nothing more to be done then this may be better in the long run than repeated failure in therapy.

Many of the problems that arise when working with older children are found with adult clients, so we suggest that the reader turns to *chapter nine* for further discussion of continuing the process of change.

CHAPTER 6
UNDERSTANDING ADULTS

Chapter 6
UNDERSTANDING ADULTS

In *chapter two*, techniques for exploring clients were outlined. Having gathered sufficient information, the therapist is in a position to formulate a transitive diagnosis. This is essentially the planning stage of therapy. The therapist seeks to find the avenues of movement along which the client may shift towards a happier future. Where other models may impose pre-emptive constructions and label disordered behaviours, personal construct therapy offers no such categories of certainty. In PCT, the diagnosis seeks to find pathways of potential change.

To this end, Kelly proposed a system of professional constructs which enable therapists to subsume their clients' personal constructs. This system provides axes or dimensions along which people may move. For example, consider the diagnostic construct *loose—tight*: if a person is construing at one end of the dimension we may predict that, as they change, they are likely to move towards the other end. Neither pole is a good or bad place to be, but rather reflects the current mode of construing and the avenues of movement open to the person when change occurs.

The examples that follow are drawn from our personal experience as therapists. Certain details have been altered or omitted to protect the identity of the clients discussed in this chapter. We would like to stress that the process of formulating a diagnosis is never quite so neat and tidy as in books. Our examples have been selected because they illustrate the points that we are trying to make and comprise just a small part of all the information gathered during diagnosis, much of which will not point so clearly to a diagnostic hypothesis. We hope that therapists will find that these examples give them an understanding of the process of formulating hypotheses and planning ways of testing these in the course of therapy.

In the event that therapists might be wondering how we settled on the specific methods for eliciting the information which has been so helpful in understanding the clients in our examples, we have to say that experience with PCT has given us the freedom to follow up hypotheses made during the early stages of therapy. While first studying PCT, we would stick fairly closely to a standard procedure of information gathering which included a self characterisation, eliciting and laddering constructs, and completing a repertory grid. Through experience, as well as discussions with our colleagues and teachers, we have developed our ability to use the process of information gathering in increasingly varying ways. We would suggest that therapists who wish to gain experience in PCT follow a similar path of learning to ourselves, and later branch out and invent their own methodologies.

The client's construction of the problem

Clients who stutter may assume that, if they say that they stutter, the therapist will automatically understand the implications of the problem and, very often, we may assume mistakenly that we do. But what does it mean to us when a person says, 'I stutter'? Probably not a lot. What we do need to know is how stuttering affects the person.

For example, Jerry tells us that he is able to run a marathon, but he cannot pick up the telephone at work for fear of stuttering. Lesley wakes up each day with a feeling of dread. She scans through the things she will have to say, looking for potentially hard words or situations that will elicit stuttering. She never sees a film that has a word beginning with /b/ in it, because she would have to lie to her friends about where she had been if they called. She never buys anything in a shop beginning with /b/. How would she answer the question, 'Where did you get that jumper?' The winter brings more fears. If her children get coughs and colds, she cannot say the name of the cough mixture, for it too begins with /b/.

Nigel tells us that people are different from animals because they can speak. Stuttering makes him feel like an animal. His self-disgust and loathing spill over his face. Another man, Jim, tells us all is well in his life except for his stuttering, and even that does not bother him overly. It comes and goes, it is a nuisance and is there anything that might help him?

We can see from these examples that stuttering means different things to different people. Probably, as therapists, we bring our own constructions to bear on how we understand the client's statement of the problem. Kelly asserts that the client's view constitutes a true formulation of the problem, but it is not the only true formulation. However it is helpful to the therapy process if we are able to accept what the client says credulously.

The client's construction of others' view of the problem

Asking the client how others view the problem provides useful additional information. With adults we may get an inkling of how important the problem is to a personal relationship. For example, Lesley, who was described above, said that her husband felt that therapy would be a waste of time; he felt that she was fine the way she was. She had made one previous attempt to have therapy, and her husband had become deeply depressed and withdrawn. We may hypothesise that their relationship is built around a theme of one person being *weak* and the other *strong*. Working with only one person would threaten the stability of their marriage.

Often stuttering causes more problems to colleagues at work than to the client. The message comes through loud and clear, 'Unless I can sort out my speech, I can forget about promotion'. On occasions this might be a useful spur to doing something about stuttering: on others, it may make clients dig their heels in and refuse to change. Finding out how others view our client's stuttering gives us an indication of the context in which the person is seeking change and the implications that change may have for the client's family.

The construction of life role

All the procedures outlined in *chapter two* are relevant here, but the self characterisation and the repertory grid in particular will give therapists an idea of how clients view their life role. We are looking for our clients' constructions of how similar or different they are to the other people in their lives.

The instructions for the self characterisation and some suggested ways of analysing the sketch are given in *chapter two*. The example that follows was written by a woman in her twenties who stutters. No attempt has been made to change the spelling and grammar of the original sketch.

(a) Example of a self characterisation

Sally is a quiet girl (woman? lady?) who lacks confidence in herself. She tends to have a pessimistic view of life which rather limits her lifestyle. I think she compensates for this by day dreaming.

She is rather shy and is almost obsessive about what other people think of her hence she dwells on any criticism/jokes etc about her. Maybe 'shy' is the wrong word to use as she can be quite outgoing at times. I think sensitive is a better description of her, infact I think she is much too sensitivity which leads to long periods of melancholy. This I think is due to the fact she is too idealistic.

She has a close group of friends and as I stated before can be very outgoing, almost an extrovert at times but tends to draw back into herself if she feels the situation is too threatening. Sometimes I get the feeling she would like to be invisible. If you were to question her friends about her or even her family they would all have different views/opinions about her personality. She adapts herself to every situation so well, so that she will be acceptable, that she often loses sight of herself.

She is a willing girl and is also very caring.

(i) Analysis of Sally's character sketch

The opening statement of the sketch gives the impression of a person who is unsure of herself in at least two ways: her lack of confidence in herself and whether she is a girl, woman or lady. Her final statement returns to the term 'girl'—perhaps she has made up her mind about her female identity? The theme 'who is Sally?' is very apparent throughout the sketch. She is not sure herself; her friends will all say different things about her and even her family cannot pin her down. She does indicate that she cares greatly about what others think of her and will try to be what others want her to be, so much so that she loses sight of herself. She wishes she were invisible at times, and seems to have discovered the next best thing: how to be a social chameleon.

She touches on a theme of constriction: her lifestyle is limited because of her tendency to be pessimistic. Her over-sensitivity to others' reactions to her and her being too idealistic leads to periods of melancholy. In contrast, her daydreams are unfettered and by implication are optimistic.

She characterises herself as quiet and shy, but later replaces 'shy' with 'sensitive'. If threatened she will retreat and would like to disappear from sight. In contrast she can be outgoing and extroverted.

Her final statement is the only one that seems unconditionally positive. It appears as if it is an afterthought, tacked on at the end without elaboration. We may hypothesise that she finds it difficult to be positive about herself, especially in the light of her uncertainty about herself. Her view of herself is largely negative and in these respects she is able to speculate on cause and effect relationships.

Sally stutters and yet has not mentioned this fact. She has told us what her problems are, and these probably flow from stuttering. The context of the sketch is by and large the social sphere. She has omitted her past, her work, her fiancé, her future. The importance of this is that interpersonal relating is probably her area of greatest difficulty. The constructs which govern her role relationships are not very helpful. She is pessimistic, too idealistic and obsessed with what others think of her. These ways of relating to others are likely to lead to feeling threatened, most especially if she picks up any signal that she is unacceptable to others. We get a sense of a cluster of constructs that is permeable at the negative end: they are good for construing bad things about herself. The more positive poles seem impermeable: unable to make sense of good things about her.

(ii) Making hypotheses

1 Sally is likely to experience guilt if she receives incontrovertible positive feedback about herself. This may lead to hostile behaviour on her part.

2 Her role constructs seem limited to construing other people's negative reactions to her. This probably causes her anxiety in situations where this type of feedback is not forthcoming, and we may guess that anxiety leads to focusing on speech, which in turn leads to stuttering.

3 She indicates areas of constriction: she has a need for certainty and probably constricts in the face of any ambiguity. She is possibly quite depressed.

4 The areas of safety for her appear to be in her daydreams and with close friends or family. We need to know more about why she is able to be outgoing.

5 Daydreaming appears to be an area of potential loose construing and may be useful to the process of change.

6 She shows very contrasting behaviour: a limited lifestyle on the one hand, with daydreams to compensate on the other; outgoing behaviour on some occasions as opposed to being quiet and withdrawn. These pathways of change are the ones that are open to her at present.

These hypotheses all have implications for therapy. Sally needs to be helped to construe herself and others in broader terms than she is able to do at present. This process will also involve finding ways of validating a more positive view of herself and we may have to render some of her current ways of construing others less permeable. At first we may have to use material from her daydreams, before we can help her to experiment with her role constructs. Even from this short character sketch we can note that she is likely to retreat in the face of anxiety. Therefore the process of change will need to be tackled slowly, making sure that Sally can make sense of each step.

(b) Example of a repertory grid

This grid was completed by Sally at about the same time as she wrote the self characterisation above. Most of the constructs in the grid echo the themes touched on in the character sketch. The graph below (*Figure 6.2*) gives an idea of how the constructs relate to each other. The correlations derive from a computer analysis of the raw data using the program called GAB, which was developed by **Bannister and Higginbotham** (1983).

From the graph we see that most of the constructs cluster around the *confident–lacking in confidence* axis. In fact the only three constructs which correlate significantly with *ambitious–unambitious* also relate significantly to confidence. What can we deduce from looking at the relationships between constructs?

Figure 6.1 Sally's grid

	Repertory Grid Sally Scale: 1–9		1 Mother	2 Father	3 Vince	4 Flora	5 As I am	6 As I'd like to be	7 Stuttering self	8 Fluent self	9 James	10 Carolyn	11 Anne	12 Kate
1	strong character	weak character	1	7	1	1	8	1	9	3	1	3	2	1
2	speaks their mind	passive	1	8	2	1	6	1	8	1	1	1	1	1
3	stubborn	easy going	1	1	2	3	5	5	8	5	1	5	5	1
4	ambitious	unambitious	1	2	1	1	3	1	8	1	2	1	1	9
5	talkative	quiet	1	7	6	2	5	2	8	2	1	3	2	1
6	very sensitive	insensitive	9	8	7	7	1	7	1	7	9	7	8	9
7	outgoing	introverted	2	8	4	2	7	2	9	7	1	3	1	3
8	very assertive	unassertive	1	8	7	1	5	1	9	7	2	2	1	1
9	very articulate	not articulate	1	5	2	2	4	1	9	2	2	1	1	2
10	confident	lacking in confidence	1	3	3	1	8	1	9	3	2	2	1	1
11	determined	undetermined	1	2	1	1	6	1	8	6	1	2	1	1
12	very friendly	unfriendly	2	2	3	1	5	2	7	4	1	4	1	4
13	calm	nervous	2	6	5	3	8	2	9	5	1	1	3	4
14	socially acceptable	socially unacceptable	1	3	2	2	5	2	9	5	2	2	1	4
15	doesn't experience fear	experiences fear	1	4	2	1	7	2	8	6	1	2	3	2

1 Sally's personal construct system is virtually monolithic. Everything is invested in one major way of looking at the world. This implies that if a person is judged as being *confident* they are also likely to be *a strong character, determined, calm, does not experience fear* and so on.

2 This also has implications for therapy. If we attempt to change Sally's way of using any of these constructs, we may be upsetting her major way of understanding people. The risks of change are enormous. Therefore the

Figure 6.2 Construct analysis

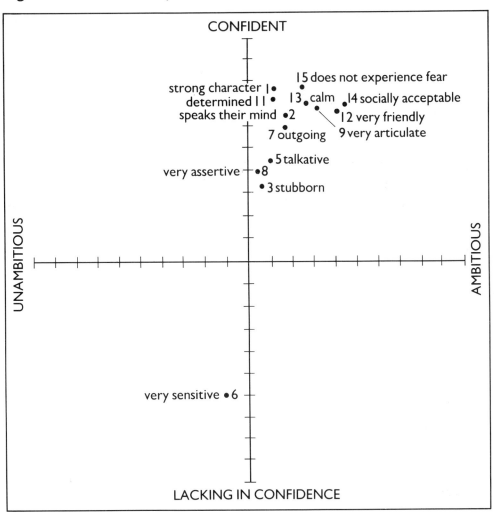

first step in therapy may need to be loosening the tight relationship between constructs, so that one does not imply the other automatically. We would look for ways of breaking the rules of her system. For instance, can she think of a person who is *very articulate* but not *calm*? We will need to teach her to speculate, something which goes against her need for certainty and predictability.

3 Many of her constructs are defined by extremes. For example, *very sensitive, very assertive, very friendly*. We also know that she uses them in an either/or fashion, not making much use of the middle ranges. It is possible that reducing the range of convenience of her constructs might be helpful, for example, *more sensitive–less sensitive*. This type of construct might encourage a looser style of construing which is also less pre-emptive.

Looking at the element analysis (*Figure 6.3*), two points immediately spring to mind:

1 Sally seems to be construing the elements *stuttering self* and *as I am* as the opposite to all the other elements in the grid.

2 The *fluent self* is unrelated to any of the other elements in the grid, and probably has little meaning for Sally.

These findings confirm everything we have discovered about Sally so far. She views herself very negatively and other people more positively. The element *as I would like to be* is right in the middle of the more positive elements, but

Figure 6.3 Element analysis

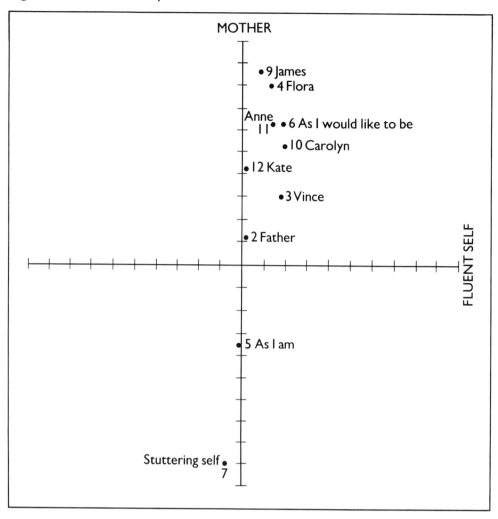

totally unrelated to *fluent self*. Change towards fluency cannot be tackled simply by learning a fluency technique. Such change will need to be accompanied by major reconstruing of self and others.

(c) Further ways of exploring personal meanings

Therapists should not feel discouraged if they do not have access to a computer. Certainly, much of the personal construct methodology can be used without resorting to a grid. Techniques of eliciting and laddering constructs or exploring implicative dilemmas can be as useful to the process of subsuming another person's construct system as doing a grid might be. It is hoped that the examples below will do justice to this assertion.

(i) Working with Sean

Sean had difficulty expressing himself, particularly in situations where he was required to say what he thought. He would often remain silent, rather than speak his mind. We decided to explore this construct further by laddering it. Sean's behaviour was governed by the non-preferred pole of the construct. Hence laddering was going to elaborate the implications of placing himself on his preferred pole. We laddered (*see chapter two, page 20*) the construct *speak up for myself—remain silent* as in the example below.

Before doing this ladder, Sean had looked at the situation solely in terms of stuttering. If he felt he was going to stutter, then he had best remain silent. Getting to the top of the ladder and seeing that speaking up for himself

speak up for myself	—	remain silent
sense of valuing self	—	feels he is not equal
can be yourself	—	do not project the 'real me' to others
less worried about others' expectations	—	makes me try too hard and I end up frustrated

actually might diminish his fears of others was very revealing and opened up new possibilities for experimenting with having his say. We can assume that the fear of stuttering and the subsequent focus on speech kept him silent and prevented him thinking through the implications of speaking up for himself.

(ii) Working with Robert

Robert was a very hostile client. During his childhood his father had been extremely strict with him and very critical of any weakness, and consequently he felt that he would always be a disappointment to his father. This motivated him to strive for perfection. He had achieved an enormous amount: a degree from Oxford, a Master's degree with distinction from a London University, a happy marriage and a good job. Yet still he felt that he was not doing well enough. His father had died, but Robert had internalised his father's critical view of himself.

The hostility manifested itself through Robert's consistent rejection of any praise or affirmation of his success from others. It seemed as if he would only accept his father's approval and, as his father was dead, we had to find a way whereby he could become more reliant on self-appraisal. The task we set him was to write his own obituary for *The Times* – the newspaper his father used to read. Unfortunately we cannot include Robert's obituary here because the details are too specific and would identify him without question. However the results of the experiment can be shared. Writing his obituary changed Robert's perception of his life in a subtle way. First, he realised that he was only 34 years old, and therefore had not yet lived as long as his father had. If he compared his achievements with those of his father at a similar age, he was doing as well, if not better than his father. Second, he realised that each person makes their own unique contribution to life on earth. He could no more mimic his father than his own son could mimic him. By looking at his son, he also understood his father's great hopes for him. Robert also wanted the best for his child, and was going to teach him to aim high, but in his own way. Third, he felt a sense of pride that he had achieved as much as he had despite his stuttering. It had not been easy, but he had managed. The way was clear to move on.

(iii) Working with Martin

Martin was feeling mildly depressed. He had moved to London to a better job, and yet was not as happy as he felt he should be. Every other sentence had the word *should* in it, which might have been a signal that he was experiencing guilt in the Kellian sense. In some way he was feeling dislodged from his core role as a happy and successful person, and did not know how to resolve the problem. Stuttering was part of the guilt pattern: 'I've had a lot of therapy: I should be fluent by now'.

He could not or would not write a self characterisation, but was prepared to list his main attributes. In discussing these, it became apparent that he had a conflict between the sort of person he needed to be at work and the sort of person he was outside work. At work, to be successful, he felt he should be very purposeful, act on what he thought was right, be independent, tackle things immediately and not be sensitive to others' opinions of him. However, outside work, he wanted to be seen as caring, kind, generous, not taking advantage of others and adhering to the old-fashioned values he had learnt at home. He felt happier and more true to self when he was this sort of person rather than the sort of person he became at work.

At work, he stuttered whenever he was called upon to be 'hard' and this left him feeling inferior and inadequate to the task. Needless to say, he was working in a high-powered business concern, not an easy context for him to be true to his core role.

(iv) Implicative dilemmas

When it came to laddering some of the constructs we had elicited, Martin frequently found that he could not decide which was his preferred pole. When this happens it is not possible to ladder the construct in the usual way, but it is possible to use the ABC method (**Tschudi**, 1977) which is described in *chapter two*. Consider the example:

a1	A caring, thinks of others' needs	a2	self-centred, does not think of others' needs
b1	B feel you are doing your best, get close to others	b2	never get as close as you would otherwise
c2	C disregard self	c1	get your own way, do your own thing, do what is right for yourself

(b1 gives the advantages of a1 and c2 gives its disadvantages. Likewise, b2 gives the disadvantages of a2 and c1 gives its advantages.)

Martin has an implicative dilemma: if he goes all out for himself he loses closeness with others, and if he tries to get close to others he ends up sacrificing his own needs. What he has to resolve is how to get close to others, but still be able to do what is right for himself. When we discussed stuttering in relation to this dilemma, Martin became aware that if he were fluent, he would expect himself to be more purposeful and achievement-orientated. Stuttering at work effectively was a way of stating 'I'm not really this kind of guy'. It resolved the guilt of seeming self-centred and maintained the *status quo*.

The ABC method is useful for fleshing out some of the risks of change. Therapy with Martin now has a focus. Instead of the problem being defined in *stuttering—fluency* terms (first order change), with the choice of technique as the obvious alternatives for therapy, the problem is now understood in terms of core role, and a different set of alternatives have become apparent (second order change). Some ideas for therapy might be:

1 Martin could change his job to one where his *caring* core role could be validated.

2 He could be helped to reconstrue *self-centred* so that he could combine being considerate with being purposeful. Perhaps being *assertive* might be a useful notion.

3 He could be helped to reconstrue fluency, so that it did not imply being *self-centred* and so on.

4 He could seek ways of validating the *caring* role in his current job: becoming a compassionate businessman.

Again, we make the point that diagnosis or exploration should lead to planning for change, rather than labelling the client.

(v) Getting at the core

With some clients all ladders seem to lead to the same superordinate constructs. In such cases, we may hypothesise that their systems are rather tightly organised, and that they have one major way of structuring their views of events. One such client was Charles. All ladders led to one of two constructs: *the need to be liked—happy with self* or *the need to be respected— happy with self*. He could understand every interaction in these terms, no matter how trivial it might seem to others. Buying a bus ticket involved respect, meeting friends at a party involved being liked, and so on. Either one of these constructs dominated every single situation he encountered. A dilemma arose for him in some situations where these two constructs conflicted with each other, producing a third choice point: *the need to be liked—the need to be respected*. For example, when he met clients at work he wanted to be both liked and respected. However, he felt that the ways he behaved in order to be liked were unworthy of respect. He would be over-friendly, ingratiating and charming. While trying to be liked he found it difficult to be decisive, stand up for his beliefs and show confidence, qualities he saw as being worthy of respect. In such situations he felt he ended up being apologetic and cringing and earned neither respect nor liking from his associates.

Where did stuttering fit in? As soon as Charles sensed that people were not responding to his friendly overtures, or that he was not worthy of respect, he would stutter and validate the prediction that he was basically unaccept-able as a person. This construct had a history: as a child he had felt rejected and unworthy. No matter how hard he tried, he failed to get his parents' attention. Perhaps stuttering got him noticed? He cannot say, but certainly the prediction that sooner or later people will reject him lies behind the extraordinary lengths he would go to in order to be liked.

Understanding this conflict of interest changes the course of therapy. We need to help Charles find alternative ways of relating to people. In the first instance, he could perhaps be asked to focus on the purpose behind mundane transactions such as shopping, or making inquiries. Instead of each situation being open to the possibility of validating or invalidating his core constructs, he could seek validation in other terms. For example, if he tried to be business-like and efficient, he could evaluate the transaction differently. Did he get what he wanted? Did he make himself understood? How long did he take to complete the transaction? and so on.

We would see this as a useful starting-point to the process of change. In the longer term he would need to find happier ways of construing himself than he was able to at present.

The therapeutic relationship

Throughout this book we have stressed the ideal therapeutic relationship as being a partnership between client and therapist. Understanding the ways in which clients may be viewing the therapist may be deduced from the constructs that have been elicited. We have found it useful to look at the client's constructs with the question in mind, 'If I used this construct to construe the therapist/therapy, how would it lead me to behave?'

In the example of Charles it soon became apparent that he had a need to be liked by the therapist. He would start off every session with a delicate inquiry as to the therapist's well-being, so much so that this behaviour was starting to obstruct the therapy process. We had to find an alternative which would not be too invalidating to Charles. The option chosen was to focus on the task at hand: not to be rejecting, but to stay professional and business-like. Examples of statements that redirected Charles to the task in hand were: 'I think we should review what we did last week, before continuing with today's agenda' and 'Let's try and finish eliciting constructs, so that we can start setting up some experiments.'

At first Charles tried to seek validation of his acceptability, seeming to have great difficulty reducing therapy to a structured transaction between himself and a therapist. In the end, he resorted to the use of a construct that had been useful to him at school and in the army: being co-operative and obedient. Again this posed problems for therapy, since obedience involves following instructions in an unquestioning way, an attitude which would mitigate against an equal partnership. One of the ways in which this was tackled was for the therapist to ask Charles for ways of solving particular problems identified during the exploratory phase. For example: 'From your self characterisation there seems to be a theme of appearance and reality. You've described your outer self with great clarity. How are we going to find out more about the inner self?' This set Charles off on a process of writing his autobiography. This would not have been the method of choice from the therapist's point of view, but was helpful in finding the roots of Charles's need to hide his real self from other people. In this case the client taught the therapist something very useful and was helped himself.

The implication of this example is that, as therapists, we need to be on the look-out for the ways in which our clients are construing us. We may not always enjoy the results of these deductions. For instance, if the client construes the therapist as an expert and behaves in a deferential manner, she may feel very uncomfortable with the powers attributed to her. However understanding the role relationship that the client is attempting to construct enables the therapist to invalidate constructs which are not useful to the client.

Many people who stutter have great difficulty construing people in broader terms than their reaction to stuttering. Very often, as clients walk into the therapy room and meet a speech therapist, they speak fluently. The therapist might be authoritarian and overbearing, but still clients speak fluently, because they predict that speech therapists are likely to be understanding and not react unfavourably to stuttering in the therapy setting. While the fluency may be useful in terms of getting through the exploratory phase more quickly, it may not be useful in the long run. The therapist has been type-cast: a therapist and nothing but a therapist. Invalidating this construction may be extremely difficult and yet it is imperative that it be invalidated if the therapist is to help the client evolve other role constructs in the course of therapy. How often have we been told by clients that a role play 'worked' because it involved ourselves, but that the same approach would not 'work' outside? In such cases we have ceased to be real people, and our ability to validate new constructions is in jeopardy.

The ways in which clients construe their therapists may involve pre-verbal constructs, which are not readily verbalisable. Such constructs are evolved before language has developed, and are useful for construing those people who meet basic needs such as providing food and shelter. Kelly points out that these constructs are not role constructs, as babies are not involved in trying to subsume the construction processes of their parents and to play a role in relation to them, but that they do influence interpersonal relationships. When the ways in which clients relate to their therapists are governed by dependency constructs, clients may behave as if their lives depended on having therapy. Therapists unwittingly may invite clients to relate to them in this way when they assume the role of the 'expert', with the implication that, as therapists, we know best what will help our clients. This may serve a valid interim goal in therapy: for example, allowing a client to depend on the therapist may help the client to verbalise and test these dependency constructs. If this is followed by formulating better ways of dealing with dependencies than the infantile way described above, the client will be able to leave therapy with a sense of autonomy and personal growth.

We need to make it clear that adults as well as children have dependencies. The differentiating factor lies in the range of convenience of these constructs: for infants, the focus may be entirely on the parents who nurture and provide for their baby; for adults, dependencies tend to be dispersed widely amongst family, friends and institutions. The scattering of dependencies enables adults to cope when threatened with the potential loss of an element subsumed by the dependency constructs. Optimally functioning adults base their dependencies on mutual understanding, which is 'the civilised alternative to the sort of infantile dependency which makes people submit to a paternalistic control in order to survive' (**Kelly**, 1955, p 671).

Trouble-shooting

When first using some of the exploratory techniques described in this book, therapists may encounter unexpected problems. For example:

■ not every client is able to verbalise their constructs;

■ sometimes the constructs that are verbalised are not understandable;

■ clients may become over-anxious about getting the verbal labels of their constructs phrased correctly;

■ sometimes rating a grid poses clients with problems because they cannot relate people to numbers;

■ some clients find writing a self characterisation very threatening and do not want to give it to the therapist.

The discussion below takes each of these points separately and attempts to account for the problems that may arise during the exploratory phase of therapy.

(a) Inability to verbalise constructs

There are a few reasons why clients may find it difficult to verbalise their constructs. Although this is a relatively rare phenomenon, some adult clients are still making extensive use of pre-verbal constructs. As these have no verbal labels, such clients may ponder triads of elements and be unable to say why any two are similar and different from the third. An example of such a client is Terry. He started stuttering at about the age of four. His mother was very distressed about this. Very soon after the onset of stuttering, his mother was diagnosed as having pre-senile dementia and was hospitalised. Terry was sent away from home to an aunt while his mother was in hospital. In his mind he connected his mother's distressed reactions to his stuttering with her illness. His subsequent banishment from home did nothing to contradict the theory that somehow or other he was to blame. From that moment on, he stopped relating to people. Later he was fetched home again, and his father gave up work to care for his very demented mother. Terry grew up thinking that if he dared to get close to anyone, somehow they would end up like his mother and so he became very withdrawn.

Therapy presented him with problems. He had never discussed any of these fears before and they were locked away in his mind in vague feelings and hunches. Trying to elicit constructs proved futile. In the first place, finding the elements from which to elicit constructs was very difficult, but once faced with these he sat in mute silence. At this stage we were unaware of his very sad story and, being new to PCT, probably persisted longer than was desirable. Bit by bit, he related the story of his life, making some of the pre-verbal issues more explicit. He talked to his father about his mother's illness and discovered that his father had not been blaming him all these years. Therapy moved incredibly slowly, catching up on a whole lifetime of experience that had been missed. The story ends with Terry being willing to relate to people, but still a very tense and sad person. We could predict that if he ever fell in love or got really close to someone, he would be faced with a huge dilemma as to how to deal with dependency issues. Meanwhile he continues to acquire social experience at a slow and steady pace.

Less extreme examples of clients who find it difficult to verbalise constructs are those who have little experience of talking about themselves. Perhaps no one has ever asked them why they think what they think; why they do what they do. Perhaps as stuttering children they did not acquire the same sort of speaking experiences that more fluent children did. Further, if other people's reactions to their stuttering is the main way in which they make sense of people, they may find it difficult to come up with other constructs.

(b) Incomprehensible constructs

Again this is an uncommon problem, which can be very perplexing when it occurs. A client called Ben gave the following verbal labels to the first construct elicited in one of the early sessions of therapy:

emotional fascist	—	*well-meaning altruist with an edge*

The strategies used for trying to uncover the meaning of this construct were laddering and pyramiding, the hypothesis being that it would be understandable at either a higher or lower level of abstraction. Laddering led to a deluge of incomprehensible terms. Pyramiding clarified the construct immediately:

inconsiderate	—	*kind and considerate*

Meaning at last! Elicitation of further constructs uncovered a possible reason for Ben's desire to obscure the meaning of his constructs. Consider the implications of:

enigmatic	—	*open to being known; can be described*

It is not too difficult to guess which pole Ben preferred.

114

Therapists who find that they do not understand a construct offered by a client need to check that their own constructs are not getting in the way of subsuming their client's way of using constructs. As in the example above, laddering or pyramiding will help to reveal the meaning and implications of constructs that are difficult to understand at first sight.

(c) Getting the verbal labels right

Clients who generally construe tightly and who may have less experience of talking about themselves, sometimes find that they cannot pinpoint the exact words of the construct. No sooner do they suggest one possible formulation than they wish to change the verbal labels of the construct. For the therapist who is struggling to subsume her client's construing, this can be very frustrating. It can also be extremely time-consuming. One of the strategies we have evolved for dealing with this problem is to suggest to clients that we press on with the elicitation, and that they take away the list of constructs during the week and change them in whatever way seems most appropriate to them.

It would seem that such clients are using the procedure to clarify their construing in verbal terms. In some cases this can be a useful and very therapeutic step; in others, it may lead to unwanted tight construing. However it is not always possible to know this in advance. If clients are agonising over the process, we would suggest that the therapist resorts to alternative methods for eliciting constructs such as conversational methods, self characterisations or other forms of writing.

(d) Difficulties with rating scales

Some clients find that using numbers to rate the various elements in their grids is difficult. They do not think in terms of numbers, but may be able to use concepts such as *more* or *less*. If this is so, ranking elements along construct dimensions may be more appropriate for them. There is a procedure for analysing ranked grids within the GAB package mentioned earlier.

Occasionally clients seem unable or unwilling to use the full scale when rating elements. They may stick cautiously to the middle ranges: for example, on a 1–7 scale, they may only use the ratings 3, 4 and 5. If all people can be rated in the middle ranges of a rating scale, what might that mean? Perhaps they are telling us that their constructs do not have great predictive efficiency. Asking such clients to rank the elements encourages them to construe the differences between their elements.

The converse can happen where clients only use the extremes of the rating scale, for example, using ratings of 1 and 7 for most of the elements. We may hypothesise that such clients view the world in a very cut and dried manner. Things are very definite and polarised. Therapy with such clients is likely to aim at loosening.

(e) Difficulties with the self characterisation

Some clients find the process of writing about themselves very threatening. They might be prepared to talk about themselves, but putting pen to paper is asking too much of them. In order to protect clients, we suggest that therapists discuss with clients how they feel about doing a self characterisation. We often suggest to clients who seem worried about it that they write a sketch which only they ever see and then try writing one which they are prepared to share with the therapist. Discussing with clients how the sketch will be used may also reduce the threats inherent in the exercise.

When clients bring a characterisation to therapy, we suggest that therapists ask them whether they want to read and discuss it during the session, whether they would like the therapist to read it during the week or whether they choose not to hand it in at all. Only on one or two occasions have clients decided not to hand in their sketches and we have respected their choice.

The process of subsuming

Therapists need to develop a system of constructs which is primarily methodological and which can subsume a wide variety of differing personal construct systems. This professional system must be verbalisable and usable and should not rival the systems of clients (**Kelly**, pp595–6).

When faced with the wealth of information that is generated by the exploratory techniques we have described, therapists may find it useful to develop a system of approach for working on this data. The following guidelines are by no means an exhaustive list of questions to put to the data, but provide a starting-point.

(a) Subsuming content

1 In what ways might these personal constructs influence the person's behaviour?
2 Are there any recurring themes among the constructs, signalling an issue of great importance to the client?
3 How are the constructs phrased? Are they descriptive of other people, or do they describe the ways in which other people relate to the client?
4 Does the person use language that seems strange, peculiar or obscure?
5 Are the constructs appropriate for the person's age?
6 Do the poles of the constructs seem to be very extreme or moderate?
7 If these constructs were my own, how would the world seem to me?

(b) Subsuming structure

1 Are the constructs pitched at an abstract or concrete level?
2 If a grid has been used, how many components are there for constructs and elements?
3 Can each component be defined in terms of a common theme?
4 Are there a lot of significant correlations, or only a few? Can this be explained?
5 Are there constructs which bridge the different components?
6 Which constructs are core constructs, and which are peripheral?

(c) Subsuming process of construing

1 Do the constructs have to do with interpersonal relating?
2 If a grid has been used, on the whole are the ratings extreme or centred around the mid-point of the scale used?
3 Are there constructs that indicate an openness to change?
4 How is self construed as compared to other elements?
5 What is the distance between self and ideal self?
6 Do any of the constructs indicate depression or withdrawal?
7 How does the person handle decision making?
8 How permeable are the constructs?

(d) Subsuming style of construing

1 Does the person use constructs pre-emptively, constellatorally or prop-ositionally?

2 Is the style of anticipation generally tight or loose?

(e) Other questions

1 What are the risks of change for the person?

2 Are there areas of aggression and active elaboration?

3 Are there areas of constriction and anxiety?

4 What will threaten this client?

5 How has this person changed over time?

6 Is the system useful for anticipating the future?

7 How does the person deal with validation and invalidation?

Many of these questions can be credited to **Landfield and Epting** (1987), and the others have emerged from our own experience.

Women as clients

Research being undertaken by Celia Levy, Louise Capstick and Suzy Wyatt to investigate how stuttering affects women is still in its very early stages. However we felt it important to share some of the questions posed by this research and to review some of the literature relating to women as clients in the hope that speech therapists would examine their ways of understanding women who stutter.

In a book entitled *The Atypical Stutterer* (St Louis, 1986) we find a chapter on women by **Silverman**. She points out that most of the research on stuttering has either excluded women or pooled their responses with those of men, so that we have no systematic body of knowledge pertaining to women who stutter. Can we use what we know of men who stutter to inform our therapy with women? There are indications, both from Silverman's research and from studies on gender as a factor in psychotherapy, that this may be unsatisfactory for women.

It has been well-established that psychotherapists have a negative stereotype of women as clients. For example, **Broverman *et al.*** investigated clinicians' ratings on the Rosenkrantz Sex-Role Questionnaire to describe a healthy, mature, socially competent adult man and woman. There was no difference in how they viewed a mentally healthy adult (sex unspecified) and a mentally healthy man. However, the description of mentally healthy women was different from that of men, portraying women as being 'more submissive, less independent, less adventurous, more easily influenced, less aggressive, less competitive, more excitable in minor crises, having their feelings more easily hurt, being more emotional, more conceited about their appearance, less objective, and disliking math and science' (**Broverman *et al*.** 1970, p4). What is considered to be ideal for men is considered to be less ideal for women, leaving women in a double-bind: they can be healthy and masculine or less healthy and feminine.

Silverman (1982) found that certified speech-language pathologists hold negative stereotypes of women who stutter, that differ from their negative stereotypes of men who stutter. It is an indictment of our profession that we hold negative stereotypes of stuttering clients at all, but that we appear to attribute additional negative qualities to women casts aspersions on our professional integrity. Although there is no comparable study in

Great Britain, **Cheasman** (1987) did find evidence of a negative view of stuttering clients as a group. Her study pointed to a sex difference in observed severity of stuttering, although therapists seemed undecided as to whether women generally were more severe or less severe than men.

Silverman (1986) points out that fewer women than men seek speech therapy help for stuttering. She hypothesises that as girls they may have had unfortunate therapy experiences, and therefore are less likely to seek treatment as adults. It is our belief that the sex ratio of clients seeking help is narrowing. More and more women are seeking therapy. In her research sample, consisting of 70 new referrals, Cheasman found that the male to female ratio was 2.7:1. What are the consequences of sex role stereotyping? **Mareck and Johnson** (1980) point out that therapists, like anyone else, are likely to be affected by the gender of their clients. **Silverman** (1986) reports that women who stutter tend to have therapy, on average, for a total of 2.8 non-consecutive years, whereas men average a total of 5.6 non-consecutive years. She hypothesises that women either respond better to therapy or leave earlier owing to bad therapy experience. We find another possible explanation in the different concept of mental health for men and women held by clinicians as described above in the study by **Broverman** *et al*. (1970). Could it be that women are discharged earlier because our standards of mental health for women are lower than for men?

Silverman indicates a tendency for women to favour a counselling approach to therapy, whereas men appear to favour learning speech controls. Therapy with adults who stutter in Britain seems to be becoming more psychologically-oriented. **Cheasman** (1987) found that a high percentage of stuttering therapists were using personal construct psychology as a back-up to traditional speech therapy techniques. Does this account for the increase in women attending therapy? Perhaps we are serving their needs better now than when almost all speech therapy involved learning fluency techniques. **Silverman and Zimmer** (1982) indicate that women may prefer individual to group therapy. Comments from clients in a group for women who stutter confirm this proposition, stating that men tend to dominate mixed groups and make them feel anxious. Our personal view is that having women in a mixed group makes the experience better for men, in that they are encouraged to express feelings by the women members of the group. It would appear that the converse may not be true for women. Being in a women-only group creates an atmosphere of equality and freedom that enables women to discuss issues that they feel might be considered to be trivial or incomprehensible by men.

In Britain most speech therapists are women. Most of our stuttering clients are men. As women, are we influenced by the importance that our society accords to the male role? Do we tend to offer therapy that meets the needs of men more readily than therapy that meets the needs of women? The time has come for us to face the challenge that is posed by women clients and to abandon the view that, because stuttering is more typical in men, women who stutter therefore must be atypical.

Professional boundaries

What constitutes a speech therapist's job? How do we decide when to refer clients to other professionals or, conversely, how do we decide that we are able to help clients resolve their problems ourselves? The answers to these questions are not very easy to generalise to all therapists, but we hope that the following points make useful guidelines:

1 **Sheehan** (1979) has perhaps been the most outspoken advocate of the stuttering therapist having additional psychological training, so that a wider range of problems can be dealt with under the aegis of speech therapy. Our own feelings coincide with this recommendation: speech therapists who wish to work with clients who stutter have a professional responsibility to seek training that will equip them with counselling and psychotherapy skills. Stuttering therapy involves attitude work, and once attitudes to do with stuttering have been discussed it is very easy for clients to progress to talking about other problems. The strategies for dealing with these difficulties may be no different from dealing with stuttering, but too often therapists lack confidence when the content of therapy moves away from speech.

2 'Listening involves a commitment . . . the clinician should always bear in mind that . . . he creates a professional obligation for himself whenever he lets a person confide in him' (**Kelly**, p955). Many therapists hold the belief that it is their duty to conduct an exhaustive interview at the start of therapy so that they can decide on the management of a particular client. From the client's perspective this process may be damaging. If at the end of such an 'interrogation' the therapist says, 'I'm afraid I can't help you, but I know a psychotherapist who may be able to help you' the client may feel that the problems raised are so overwhelming that there is little hope of resolution. Further, the prospect of another such interview might be daunting. Giving a complete account of 'the problem' may leave a client feeling very vulnerable and exposed. Here is a person who knows so much about them, and yet they may never meet again. Kelly recommends that we allow clients to confide in us 'only to the extent that we are willing to accept responsibility for seeing that the venture works out well for the person who confides' (p955).

Where does this leave a newly qualified therapist, or an experienced therapist who wishes to work with stuttering clients for the first time? One of the best ways of acquiring experience in stuttering therapy is by doing it. But the venture should not stop at this point. In order to learn from such experience, the therapist needs to construe it and consider the implications for the rest of her personal construct system. There are at least two avenues open to therapists: first, to write detailed case-notes which involve making predictions at the end of sessions as to what the client may do with the content of the session during the week, and second, to arrange supervision with a more experienced therapist. Of course, these suggestions are not mutually exclusive.

When first starting out, therapists might wish to restrict their therapy to speech-related issues. If referrals are made to other professionals, the speech therapist can learn much from asking them how they have managed the client. As the therapist gains an increasing understanding of the nature of stuttering and its related problems, she may be more willing to explore new territory with clients. It is at this point that support from a supervisor is most crucial and useful.

Very often, at the start of therapy, the clients talk only about speech problems. As therapy progresses and they come to trust the therapist's judgements, they may wish to include other issues. For this reason it is impossible to judge at an initial interview exactly what steps will need to be taken with respect to any one client's problems. Diagnosis and therapy do not separate into neat categories. For example, Sean, who was described on page 108, started off therapy on an intensive course. He did extremely well, and left to further his studies. About four years later he returned saying that he felt he was not achieving his full potential and was interested in having some personal construct therapy. Again this went extremely well. He changed jobs, started having serious relationships with women, bought a car, moved house and started reading newspapers so that he would have informed opinions when discussing political issues with his friends. He felt as if he was fulfilling his potential.

Therapy stopped for about three months, after which he returned to discuss further problems he was having. For the first time he started to talk about his family relationships and how difficult he was finding it to go against the very strict upbringing he had had. His parents were due to visit him and he knew they would be disappointed in him: the fact that he drank alcohol, did not go to church every Sunday, and so on, was going to be criticised. He did not know how to handle letting his parents know that he had a right to choose for himself. It is likely that these problems were present at the start of therapy, but took something like five years to surface. They have been resolved now, and Sean is actively and enthusiastically living a busy life. He visited recently, six months after the last contact, to say that he had torn up his self characterisation of 18 months previously: it no longer related to the present and he recognised that he had changed.

Conclusion

The aim of this chapter has been to help therapists understand more about factors underlying stuttering and to suggest possible strategies for hypothesis making and testing in the planning phase of therapy. We feel that therapy with adults who stutter needs to take account of individual differences, and that, when therapists become more involved in the psychological factors underlying stuttering, these differences will become apparent. Through our cumulative experience of working with adults, we are prepared to assert that the mechanical manipulation of speech production only addresses one aspect of the problems of people who stutter. Only occasionally is this the sole problem.

CHAPTER 7
THERAPY
WITH ADULTS

Chapter 7
THERAPY
WITH ADULTS

We have divided our discussion of stuttering therapy with adults into five phases:

- The exploratory phase
- The planning phase
- A pre-technique phase
- Direct speech work
- Continuing the process of change

Although we recommend that therapists work through all phases, the length of each phase may vary for different clients. Not all clients will need all five phases; for example, people with more interiorised stuttering may require little or no direct speech work. Some clients make changes in their speech as a result of changing their ways of thinking about themselves, and consequently do not require formal work on speech modification. Occasionally, different therapists may be involved in the different phases, as happens when a client is referred to another agency for an intensive course, but requires therapy before and after the course.

In this chapter we propose to deal with the pre-technique and direct speech work phases. The other phases are deal with in *chapters two, six* and *nine*. A selection of activities is presented in *chapter eight* for use with groups. Most of these will be of use in the two phases of therapy under discussion in this chapter. Therapists may have to adapt the activities to suit individual therapy if this is the approach of choice.

Pre-technique work

At the 1986 conference called *Working with Stuttering in Britain*, Cheasman raised an important issue for speech therapists, asking to what extent we attempt to help our clients become 'better' clients. This section aims to address this issue and to provide some ways that therapists might help their clients to make good use of therapy: a skill which we believe can be learned and which enables clients to become their own therapists in the long term.

When an adult asks a speech therapist for help it is unlikely that this will be the first time that they have seen a speech therapist. Past experiences of speech therapy do not imply necessarily that the client is able to make maximum use of what is offered. In fact the contrary may be the case: if therapy has been unhelpful in the past, the client may feel quite sceptical about how helpful it will be this time round. This may affect their attitude to therapy and the subsequent commitment that they are prepared to make.

(a) Resistance

Many behaviour therapists include sections or chapters on motivation in their stuttering programmes. Selecting appropriate reinforcers, signing of contracts, token economies and so on are all part of this discussion. What does personal construct theory have to say about the *motivation—resistance* construct?

The answer to this question may present some therapists with an unforeseen problem. This familiar construct does not exist within PCT. We have no reason to doubt clients when they say they want to change. The onus is on the therapist to find ways of helping clients to do so. Likewise, when clients are not doing the things we expect them to do in order to change, we cannot conveniently describe their lack of co-operation as 'resistance', but have to look to concepts such as 'threat' and 'anxiety' for the answer. It is possible that therapy may threaten clients or make them feel so uncertain that they are unable to venture forward. The only way to preserve the structure on which they depend is to fail to do what the therapist wants them to do. Again, the burden of responsibility lies with the therapist, who must find ways of making change manageable for her clients.

We hypothesise that if therapists have been thorough in collecting information and planning therapy, the risks of change for the client will have been assessed. The strategies for tackling the problems should flow from hypotheses formulated during these phases. However it is possible that clients may reveal deeper troubles when they start to find change difficult. Therapy may need to involve further exploration of such issues when they are raised. Although therapy should always be challenging for clients, we subscribe to the point of view that clients should not be pushed into a corner from which there is no way out. The therapist bears the responsibility for making change possible for clients by virtue of her understanding of their personal construct systems.

(b) Dealing with an immediate crisis

Very often clients seek help urgently because they are facing a situation which they fear. Examples of this include wedding speeches, giving a presentation at work, involvement in a radio or TV programme and so on. Clients' expectations may be very unrealistic: they would like to be fluent, but they have only a few weeks in which to achieve this goal.

It is important to respond to such requests for help, even though the logistics of arranging a few sessions at short notice may be difficult. The expectation of help may have a calming effect in itself. In such circumstances we make it clear to clients that we cannot grant their wish for total fluency on the day, but that we are prepared to help them to prepare for the event and support them through it. The ways in which we try to help are as follows:

- Exploring the consequences of stuttering in the situation: *How is your audience going to react if you stutter? How do you know? What is the worst possible consequence of stuttering? Is this likely to happen? What are the consequences of not being very good at giving speeches? What things are you good at?*

- Giving permission to stutter: this involves explaining the fact that if a person tries to stutter, very often they cannot. *Choosing to stutter might be easier than living with the uncertainty of wondering if you will be fluent.*

- Can stuttering be used to good effect? *Acknowledging that you stutter, making a stuttering joke, obviously changing a word to confuse the audience, are some ways of not denying your stuttering.*

■ Rehearsing and preparing: ensuring that the client is well-prepared, has notes on cards, has an idea of how to stand, some tips on breathing and relaxation, are all helpful and take some of the focus off speech. Use of video- or tape-recorders is useful.

■ Setting up realistic aims for the situation: too many clients have expectations of giving the best talk in the world. They expect that they should be able to be funny, clever, fluent and so on, when this is clearly unrealistic. We introduce the idea that if a person who stutters gives a talk, that is admirable in itself and worthy of respect regardless of the level of fluency, which is only one criterion by which success can be judged.

■ Setting up a meeting with another client who has 'survived' such an event may be helpful.

■ Reducing the importance of the situation to just one event in a lifetime of events may make it somewhat more manageable. For example, with a client who was dreading his wedding speech, we focused on the importance of the marriage relative to the importance of the speech.

(c) Reviewing past therapy experiences

As mentioned earlier, most adults who come for therapy have some past experiences of stuttering therapy. We need to find out how they view these experiences. Stuttering leads many people to feel that they are failures: every time they open their mouths to speak they try not to stutter, and almost always fail. Therapy may reinforce the notion that they are failures. How else can they account for relapse? How do they explain their inability to use the techniques outside therapy which generate fluency in the clinic? If they had a high regard for their past therapists, the only possible explanation for their inability to maintain fluency is that somehow *they* have failed. Such clients may be very discouraged.

Other clients have an alternative perspective, which is also a less than helpful approach to therapy. They attribute the lack of success of previous therapy to the poor skills of the therapist. While we do not wish to deny that they may be right, the key issue here is the clients' view of who bears responsibility for the outcome of therapy. Such clients tend to shop around for therapists, each time hopeful that therapy will work. While they may feel less discouraged at failure, their approach to therapy goes something like, 'Let's see what this one can do'.

Reviewing past experiences of therapy enables therapists to challenge some of the implicit assumptions that clients bring to therapy. Personal construct theory offers a useful way of making sense of experience. The questions that follow fit into what Kelly called *controlled elaboration*, which is discussed under interviewing skills in the final chapter.

■ From your past experiences of therapy, what were the most useful things you learned about yourself?

■ What did you find easiest to change about yourself?

■ What did you find hardest to change about yourself?

■ What is your theory about why you were unable to maintain fluency?

■ What did your friends and family think caused your stuttering to increase again?

■ What steps did you take when you felt your speech was deteriorating?

■ With hindsight, what might have helped?

■ If you had taken these steps, how might things have been different today?

124

- What mistakes did you make in the way you made use of therapy before?
- What mistakes did the therapists make?
- How would things be different if these mistakes had not been made?
- How do you think your approach to therapy now is different from your approach in the past?
- What are you going to do if you feel your therapist is not getting therapy right?
- What are you going to do if you feel you are not working as hard as you would like to?

During this discussion the therapist is likely to be more helpful and learn more if she is able to listen credulously. These questions are geared to helping clients make use of past therapy by exploring the alternatives. Clients may find it difficult and possibly threatening to answer some of the questions and may need time to think about them.

(d) The experimental approach to stuttering therapy

Teaching clients how to experiment sets the stage for change. It enables clients to test newly formed constructs and collect evidence in a structured fashion. In the early stages of therapy we suggest that therapists ask clients to experiment with changing some behaviour that has nothing to do with speech control. There may be less risk attached to such change, and clients can learn about the process without having a vested interest in the outcome of the experiment. **Epting and Amerikaner** (1980) provide us with a breakdown of the experimental process into five successive steps:

1 *Anticipation:* the forecasting of events. For example, we might ask John to predict what would happen if he used people's names when he spoke to them. How would he feel? How would others feel and react? What would the difference be between using people's names and not using people's names? **Epting and Amerikaner** (p69) suggest that clients use the following sentences to formulate hypotheses:

- I predict that if I *use people's names* then my (roommate, mother, girlfriend, etc) will respond to me by *being more friendly*.
- If I try *using people's names* the difficulties I anticipate are *that I might stutter more*.
- When I change my behaviour in this way (or during the time I am attempting to change my behaviour), I will probably feel *a bit self-conscious*.
- When I successfully complete this change, the outcome in terms of my personal and interpersonal life will include *feeling more like other people*.

2 *Investment:* or the readiness to become involved in an experiment. Here John accepts that there are alternative ways of approaching the situation and prepares to enter the situation with the question in mind, 'What will happen if I use Joe's name when I speak to him?' The client needs to be aware of exactly what is being tested. All too often stuttering clients enlarge the experiment and test their self-worth when conducting what seems, in the therapist's eyes, to be a tightly defined experiment. Encapsulating the experiment by defining the constructs on which it is based and specifying the implications of the outcome will help clients to make the appropriate investment in testing their hypotheses.

3 *Encounter:* or commitment to the experiment. Here clients test their

predictions by engaging in the experiment. In order to learn from it, clients must be open to the experience and try not to distort events. In our example, John will try to use people's names in a natural way. If he were to use them every few words, he would be distorting events, probably to prove a point: he would not be open and questioning.

4 **Confirmation and disconfirmation:** assessing the results of the experiment. John is asked to review the consequences of using people's names. Did the predictions come off or not? Did he feel the way he thought he would feel? Did others react in the way he predicted? What was the difference between using names and not using them? If he was unable to use names, his predictions were probably innappropriate. It is not as important to be right as to be able to make good use of this process of construing.

5 **Constructive revision:** making sense of the implications of the experiment. If John had been able to use people's names, and his predictions had been borne out, what does this mean to him? What previously used constructs are rendered useless as a result of this experience? Some spring-cleaning may be necessary if the new constructs are to be incorporated into his system. Other therapeutic models speak of growth when describing this process: **Kelly** (1980) speaks of optimal functioning.

(e) Attitudes to fluency

Before commencing a course of speech modification work it may be useful to explore with clients their attitudes to the different speech techniques and to fluency itself. **Stewart** (1987a) believes that improvement in therapy is more likely in clients who have a positive attitude to fluent speech and a high intention to use a fluency technique. Her work relates only to attitudes to fluency techniques and not to block modification techniques, but we assume that the same principles could apply to either approach. Stewart is currently engaged in research to test her hypothesis. After a thorough assessment of her clients' attitudes to fluency and intentions to use prolonged speech, clients are given 12 sessions of group therapy chiefly aimed at elaborating ideas about fluency. Without having to commit themselves to the technique, clients are given the opportunity to take a look at the product, to speculate on its impact on their lives, and the chance to revise their constructs about fluency control. Although her research is not complete, she is very encouraged by assessments at the one-year stage: clients who completed the 'attitude to fluency programme' have changed their attitudes and maintained fluency at a significantly higher level than those who only learned the technique (**Stewart**, 1987b).

Because she is conducting research, her clients are not given the choice as to whether or not to learn prolonged speech, but this is certainly a possibility in therapy not geared to research. Where clients discover during the preparatory work that fluency via a control technique is not what they want, much time and effort can be spared by not proceeding with this approach.

Stewart makes the valid point that attitudes and behaviour are inextricably linked to each other. Change in behaviour will not come about unless there is a corresponding change in attitude. Change in attitude is only confirmed when we conduct new behavioural experiments and examine the consequences of our actions. Approaches to therapy that reduce the person either to their behaviour or to their attitudes do not serve their long-term interests.

(f) Bibliotherapy

Giving clients books to read to increase their knowledge about the process of change, stuttering, and communication in general may be very helpful. We suggest that therapists read for themselves the books listed below in order to assess their relevance and complexity before recommending them to clients. The list comprises books about stuttering, assertiveness, depression and personal construct theory. We leave to therapists the responsibility for selecting appropriately for their clients.

Fraser M, *Self Therapy for the Stutterer*, Speech Foundation of America, Tennessee, 1987.

Byrne R, *Let's Talk about Stammering*, George Allen & Unwin, London, 1983.

Murray F, *A Stutterer's Story*, Interstate Printers and Publishers, Danville, Ill, 1980.

Dickson A, *A Woman in your own Right*, Quartet Books, London, 1982.

Cox G and **Dainow S,** *Making the Most of Yourself*, Sheldon Press, London, 1985.

Alberti RE and **Emmons ML,** *Your Perfect Right,* Impact Publishers, California, 1970.

Rowe D, *Depression: The Way out of Your Prison*, Routledge & Kegan Paul, London, 1983.

Bannister D and **Fransella F,** *Inquiring Man*, Croom Helm, London, 1986.

(g) Meeting clients who are in the final stages of therapy

To reduce anxiety and to structure their anticipations of therapy, it may be useful to introduce clients in the early stages to those who are in the final stages of therapy. This encourages a more realistic approach in that the time scale of therapy, the ups and downs along the way and the amount of work involved can be described. Questions about the value of therapy and how and why it has helped can be discussed.

(h) Involving family, colleagues & friends

If clients are to make changes in their lives, it may be important to assess the extent to which they will be supported during the process of change. Encouraging realistic expectations from those close to our clients may be very helpful. Sometimes wives or husbands want to be involved in their partner's therapy. Any involvement of outsiders needs to be discussed with the clients first, and is not always necessary. Very often clients may wish to tell their associates about therapy in outside contexts, rather than have them come into the hospital, clinic or centre.

Many clients have found it useful to talk to colleagues at work about therapy before they go on an intensive course. This reduces the threats of other people's expectations when they return to work. Discussing the fact that stuttering cannot be cured, and that therapy is a long-term commitment with ups and downs along the way, gives associates an idea of what is involved.

(i) The therapeutic relationship

Discussions about the nature of the therapeutic relationship can be very instructive for clients who are not quite sure what to make of a speech therapist. Is she like a doctor? Is she going to be a friend? Is she like a teacher? Will she take responsibility for the problem? How formal or informal should the relationship be? Why does she not answer questions about herself?

We cannot expect clients to conform to our perception of the ideal client role unless we are prepared to engage in discussions about therapy and how the roles of expert on the process of change and expert on self match up.

Summary

Once clients have been through the exploratory phase and some pre-technique discussions they should be ready to proceed to speech modification itself. The transition between these phases needs to be made in a smooth and logical way. For clients, learning to change the way they speak should be no different now from learning to change any aspect of their behaviour and way of thinking.

Direct speech work

Stuttering therapy appears to be in a transitional phase. **Cheasman** (1987) conducted a survey on British speech therapists' views on stuttering therapy and found that the majority of therapists were using more than one approach, with a parallel trend towards subgrouping clients. The implication of this is that, currently, therapists seem concerned to match their approach to the needs of the client, reversing the previous situation where clients were offered whatever approach was 'fashionable'. Although this tendency augurs well for clients, therapists are now faced with the problem of specifying the criteria used to choose an approach for a client. Past successes and failures in therapy may serve as pointers, but because of the long-term nature of stuttering therapy, collecting information in this way is a very slow process. Even though it is evident that therapists are making choices when they select a therapeutic approach for a client, we surmise that these choices are based on clinical hunches which may or may not be valid.

We would like to recommend an interim approach to the issue of selection until such time as we have more useful criteria on which to base our decisions. For too long we have approached therapy as if we have only one chance when deciding on an approach, and once committed to that choice we have to see it through. However, if we view stuttering therapy as a series of successive choices based on information accumulated over time, we will be less afraid of making the wrong decision. **Byrne** (1987) has described her approach to very severe stuttering in adults in these terms. Based on the changing needs of her clients, she may alter the theoretical rationale of her approach. She cautions therapists to make the change smooth and logical for clients, but otherwise can find no drawback to varying her approach within one course of therapy. If anything, clients are equipped with 'extra weapons' to deal with problems.

We feel that the way forward is to structure our anticipations within a sound theoretical framework. If we have a theory about people, then we will have some notion of why people stutter. If we have a theory about how people change, we will have some ideas about how to facilitate that change. As we have indicated in the first chapter, personal construct theory has provided us with just such a framework and we would like to invite our readers to join us in taking a look at speech change from this perspective.

In earlier chapters we outlined our approach to the exploration of the person who stutters. Equipped with information about the whole person, the therapist will be in a position to make hypotheses to be tested in the context of therapy. Information about speech and stuttering is less helpful than an understanding of how the person views their problem, what they would like from therapy, what they do not want to happen, how they approach change in other contexts, what they have tried to do about their speech before, what they make of the results of such efforts and what they believe needs to be done at this stage. Such questions encourage the client to speculate and to share responsibility for solving the problem with the therapist.

We suggest the Kellian model for the therapeutic relationship, where client and therapist are co-experimenters, jointly exploring what works and what does not. Hypotheses and experiments are set up in partnership: the evidence is evaluated and reviewed together, and decisions as to how to proceed are put into effect. The therapist brings to therapy knowledge and ideas of what has helped other people: she knows how to set up experiments and facilitate change. Clients know much about themselves; they know what they want, what has helped and what has not helped. Neither can succeed in bringing about change without the other's expertise and contribution. Therapy becomes a joint venture (**Kelly**, 1955).

Are these ideas workable when drawing on techniques that emanate from a more behavioural model? We believe they are. A personal construct therapist bases her choice of techniques on a more superordinate understanding of the client, but is free to draw upon any techniques from other models. How techniques are taught, and how therapy is evaluated will differ from the source model.

Currently, there are two main approaches to changing the speech patterns of adults who stutter: the *stutter-more-fluently approach* and the *speak-more-fluently approach* (**Gregory**, 1979). Some therapists combine the two models (**Cheasman**, 1983). In our opinion the stutter-more-fluently approaches offer a wider range of possibilities to clients, chiefly because attitude change is seen as basic to long-term change. The fluency approaches also offer much to clients, but may need to be backed up by work on reconstruing to ensure maintenance of fluency (**Evesham**, 1987). We see our primary role as creating movement in our clients' construct systems during therapy. How the client construes stuttering and change will determine the choice of therapeutic style and use of techniques.

For example, most fluency techniques involve slowing down speech. If for any reason clients have the idea that slowing down sounds strange, then they are less likely to use the technique in situations where they want to sound as natural as possible, even if it means stuttering. With such clients there are two choices: first, the therapist could help them to revise their attitude to slow speech or, second, an alternative approach could be used, such as easy stuttering.

The main therapy approaches to modifying the speech of adults who stutter will now be described briefly. These include prolonged speech, block modification therapy and avoidance reduction therapy. Therapists have the option of teaching these as a package, or of introducing their clients to the experimental approach described above. If the latter path is chosen, therapists will need to design a series of meaningful experiments for their clients, covering each of the relevant aspects of the techniques and possibly including others not mentioned below. This choice is challenging and risky for the therapist. It involves a personal investment in therapy not called for in the 'package' approach, where the therapists may legitimately blame the technique rather than their own skills if they fail.

(a) Prolonged speech: a speak-more-fluently approach

This approach aims to replace stuttered speech with fluent speech by teaching a technique called prolonged or smooth speech (**Perkins**, 1979). Usually it is administered within an operant framework, and fluent speech is shaped from a very slow and prolonged rate (at 40 syllables per minute) to normal sounding speech (at 180–220 spm). Reinforcement is contingent upon the correct response, and may vary from verbal praise to tokens. The parameters of the prolonged speech technique are exaggerations of the features of fluent speech, and each can be considered to be a fluency technique in its own right. If the 'package' option is chosen, therapists might like to consider that some features of the technique are more useful than others to different clients.

1 *Prolongation* is the key feature of the technique. **Perkins** (1979) is convinced that slowing down the articulatory rate is more effective than merely slowing down the word rate. The client is taught to speak at very slow rates of 40–50 syllables per minute. Gradually, the speaking rate is increased in steps of 10 to 20 spm until normal speeds are reached. **Evesham** (1987) suggests that each stage be numbered stage one, stage two and so on. Her clients are not required to know the exact rate for each stage, but are required to be able to produce it or monitor it in others' speech.

2 *Flow* is the next feature to be taught. Words run together until the appropriate juncture for pausing and breathing. Many adults who stutter are surprised to learn that flow is part of fluent speech. They have been focused on the first sounds of words for so long, that they have forgotten that spoken language flows like a river of sound.

3 *Pausing* at the ends of phrases, or whenever breath is required, is one of the more difficult and yet important parts of the technique. Most people who stutter feel compelled to keep going once they have started, as if they have to make up for time lost while blocking. Others want to try and get as many words as possible said before they block. Whatever the case, many people find that pausing is very difficult and somehow unnatural. In the early stages of prolonged speech frequent pausing is necessary, often at meaningless points in a sentence. Later, pauses help to structure meaning by breaking up sentences into phrases. Combining pausing with breathing may help clients feel less threatened by the break in the flow, and may serve to relax them.

4 *Soft contacts* are taught as a way of reducing articulatory tension and pressure. Clients are required to make sounds gently, giving speech a slightly slurred quality at the slower rates. As rates increase, the soft contacts should be modified to as near normal as possible, but may be retained on difficult sounds.

5 *Easy onsets* are sometimes taught to help clients who block at the start of speaking, owing to laryngeal tension. Slowly sighing, then gently approx-imating the vocal cords and articulating the first sound may help people who have excessive glottal tension.

There are many variations in the way prolonged speech is taught. Some therapists introduce all the features of prolonged speech simultaneously. However **Boberg and Kully** (1985) first establish rate control before introducing any other modifications to speech. They also stress the import-ance of teaching clients about speech production, so that they have a better chance of learning to monitor their technique. The type of reinforcement varies from one therapist to the next. Some therapists use a token economy (**Evesham**, 1987), while others use verbal praise. **Shames and Florance**

(1980) reward their clients with unmonitored speech, which they believe helps them to maintain control in the long term. For every period of time where the technique is used successfully clients may have a corresponding period of time where they do not use the technique.

Similarities across most programmes include the commitment to ideas drawn from behaviour therapy: establishment, transfer and maintenance phases form part of many programmes. There is also agreement that speech should sound normal if clients are to use the technique in situations outside therapy (**Perkins**, 1979).

If a Kellian approach were to be used to modify speech in this way, therapy would have a very different complexion indeed. Prolonged speech would not be taught as a 'technique', but as a set of skills 'to be developed and made their own' (**Dalton**, 1987a, p57). Clients would check their predictions in relation to each feature of the technique and then begin to engage in experiments outside therapy almost immediately, eliminating the establishment, transfer and maintenance phases typical of behaviour therapy. The kind of speech aimed at must relate closely to the way in which clients wish to come across, or it is unlikely to be used. Speech change needs to be personalised, and teaching prolonged speech as a technique keeps it external and 'other than self'. Using a technique may feel like acting a part; using a skill requires involvement and commitment to the enterprise.

A personal construct therapy approach would be geared more towards helping clients to elaborate the meaningfulness of fluency thus acquired than to teaching and practising a control technique. Advocates of the 'practice makes perfect' approach would argue that, until responses are relatively stable in the clinic, there would be no transfer to the outside. Kellian therapists would counter by arguing that unless the changes were made meaningful to the person in some way, long-term change would not be possible. Superficial changes in speech production are akin to papering over the cracks, unless supported by reconstruction.

(b) The elaboration of fluency

Fransella (1972) validated her hypothesis that adults who stutter have a poorly elaborated system of constructs to do with themselves as fluent speakers. She posed a challenge to therapists, asserting that relapse is less likely in clients who are able to construe from a fluent speaker's point of view. **Evesham and Fransella** (1985) tested this by helping clients who had established fluency via prolonged speech to elaborate the meaningfulness of this fluency. They found that relapse was significantly reduced in clients who had had personal construct therapy as well as prolonged speech.

Helping clients to construe fluency is *not* a technique and requires some understanding of the theoretical concepts underlying personal construct psychology. The following example will give readers a feel for the process. Martin arrived for his session very pleased with himself. He had successfully (that is, fluently) done a presentation on a management course. The following dialogue ensued:

Therapist: Did you predict that you were going to speak fluently?
Martin: God no! I was as scared as hell!
Therapist: Why do you think you were fluent then?
Martin: I don't know . . . it was just numbers and things.
Therapist: I'm not sure I'm with you.
Martin: Well, it wasn't very important stuff. I just had to say what I thought. I could have been wrong and no one would have known the difference.

Therapist: So the content was less important . . .

Martin: Yes. It was pretty boring stuff.

Therapist: Describe the situation to me. How many people were present? How did they react to your talk?

Martin: Oh, fine. They had to listen.

Therapist: Surely you're not telling me that they listened because they had to! No one has ever made me listen that way. How could you tell that they were listening?

Martin: They were looking at me.

Therapist: What were their expressions like?

Martin: Fairly blank, mostly. But I felt they were listening.

Therapist: Was there anything else?

Martin: Nods, occasionally . . . I can't say I noticed much more.

Therapist: How do you think they saw you?

Martin: I haven't a clue.

Therapist: After we've got so far! Come on, shut your eyes and think back. See yourself standing up front giving the talk. Now sit in the audience and watch. What do you make of Martin? How is he doing?

Martin: OK, really. Nothing out of the ordinary. I don't think he's making any impression really.

Therapist: I don't buy that.

Martin: Well, I can't say. I'm sorry.

Therapist: Would you say that you seemed poised?

Martin: Not really ... I was very nervous, but I think I hid that well. Perhaps I seemed to cope OK with the task. I didn't have any problems, really. I just got up and did it.

Therapist: Efficiently?

Martin: Yes.

From quite a persistent series of questions, Martin began bit by bit to elaborate the experience. This was one of the first times he had been quizzed so thoroughly, and he became quite irritated, not seeing the point and puzzled that the answers should be so important. Many opportunities in that conversation became apparent after the event, such as finding out more about why it was easy for him to be fluent when saying unimportant things and not, by implication, when saying important things. However one line of inquiry was chosen and followed through. The experience could no longer be construed as 'the absence of stuttering' but was supported by some tenuous constructs that would need further elaboration and testing in future sessions.

(c) Block modification therapy: a stutter-more-fluently approach

The aims of this approach are twofold: first, to change attitudes and feelings linked with stuttering, and second, to modify stuttering towards an easier, simpler pattern. **Van Riper** (1973) is the chief advocate of this approach. Fluency is deemed to be the by-product of successful therapy, not its main aim. His programme of therapy is divided into five phases, each of which is outlined below.

1 *Identification:* This phase of therapy helps the client to describe both the stuttering feelings and behaviours that need changing before free communication can be achieved. In *chapter eight* ways of tackling identification are described. The identification process aims to demonstrate to clients that:

- stuttering is something they do, rather than something that happens to them;
- stuttering is not random, but an integrated, recurring pattern of speech;
- awareness of what they do can lead to change;
- confronting stuttering makes them feel less sensitive about it.

During this phase curiosity is more important than behavioural change. Much of the identification of stuttering takes place outside therapy, bridging the gap right away between the therapy room and the 'real world' outside.

2 *Desensitisation:* The aim is to begin to change feelings and reactions associated with stuttering. Through various activities such as learning to tolerate silences, voluntary stuttering, faked stuttering, keeping eye contact, resisting time pressure and so on, clients learn to react less negatively to stuttering. **Van Riper** (1973) uses key words such as 'calming' and 'toughening' to describe what he means by desensitisation. Like all advocates of the stutter-more-fluently approaches, he shares the belief that stuttering stops when desensitisation is complete. In a course of therapy we can only hope to begin to reduce some of the negative feelings associated with stuttering, and to provide clients with strategies for continuing to desensitise themselves in the future.

3 *Variation:* This part of therapy involves experimenting with change: attempting to be different, rather than to correct behaviour. Both speech and non-speech behaviours can be varied by omitting, adding, contrasting or diminishing them. Discussions focus on what it is like to change, how easy/difficult it is to maintain change and what choices we have. Van Riper's ideas about change are very similar to those of Kelly, to whom he actually refers in this section.

4 *Modification:* The aim of this phase is to produce easy or fluent stuttering. This goal is achieved by working through each of the following three sub-phases:

- Post-block correction: First the client learns to pause after completing a stuttered word; then, after finishing a stuttered word, to pantomime the key features of the stuttering behaviour and finally, after a stuttered word, the client pauses and then repeats the word in a slow, modified fashion. In each stage, the pause after stuttering is very important and can be used to calm down and plan ahead. Post-block correction sets up the model for easier and more fluent stuttering.

- In-block correction: During the actual block, the client modifies the stutter by controlling the release of the sound. If this is not possible, the client may use post-block correction.

- Pre-block correction: When stuttering is anticipated, the person prepares to say the word in an easy and smooth manner. If this is not possible, or if stuttering had not been anticipated, the client may use in-block correction.

Because the person is calmer and more able to tolerate stuttering following working through the desensitisation phase, it is easier to work directly with stuttering, producing an easier and more fluent sounding result.

5 *Stabilisation:* This phase directs itself to entrenching the newly acquired responses: learning to resist the old triggers of stuttering and to cope psychologically with the new style of speech. Various techniques are used: to stabilise proprioceptive monitoring, Van Riper draws on ideas from

servotheory such as shadowing, delayed auditory feedback, choral reading and the use of an electrolarynx. Counselling and psychotherapy techniques are used to help clients accept the implications of change.

Only the barest outline of Van Riper's approach has been given above. If therapists are interested in pursuing his ideas, there is no substitute for reading Van Riper in his own inimitable style.

(d) Avoidance-reduction therapy: a stutter-more-fluently approach

Sheehan and Sheehan (1984, p147) subscribe to the view that 'stuttering is perpetuated by successful avoidance and suppression of outward stuttering behaviour'. Although Sheehan's approach falls well within the stutter-more-fluently camp, he is at odds with Van Riper, rejecting the need for any control techniques, such as block modification. To Sheehan, avoidance-reduction is the key to a successful outcome. If people can stop avoiding, stop pretending and covering up stuttering from their listeners, they have the chance to recover from stuttering. Sheehan divides his therapy into the following stages:

1 *The self-acceptance phase* begins with the development of eye contact. Clients are urged to establish eye contact before speaking, even if listeners are unable to maintain eye contact. During this phase clients discuss stuttering and therapy with as many people as possible. Feelings are identified and confronted. Information about stuttering and the process of therapy is provided to give clients landmarks against which to plot their progress.

2 *Monitoring and exploring* stuttering help clients to understand what they do when they stutter. To this end, **Sheehan** (1975) has devised a 'Speech Pattern Checklist' which clients use to identify the various overt aspects of stuttering. It focuses on different ways of suppressing stuttering such as avoidance, postponement and the use of starters. The questionnaire is phrased in such a way that clients are forced to take responsibility for stuttering. For example, 'I give up when I have difficulty'; 'I substitute words', and so on. Clients monitor their use of each of these crutches in different speaking situations outside therapy. The object here is not to bring about change, but to increase awareness and a recognition of who is responsible for stuttering. This is very similar to Van Riper's 'identification' phase.

3 *The initiative phase* encourages people to tackle feared situations and words rather than letting them happen. This is where Sheehan encourages people to 'approach' rather than 'avoid' speaking. Ways of judging successes and failures are provided: for example, open stuttering, eye contact, monitoring of speech and talking about stuttering are all considered to be speech successes, while substituting words, losing eye contact and trying to talk fluently at any cost are considered to be speech failures.

4 *The modification phase* is geared towards exposing the hidden parts of stuttering, rather than trying to sound better in the ears of the listener. Voluntary stuttering in the form of a prolongation or slide is used. Clients try to stutter openly and easily on real blocks, moving forward and reducing struggle. Some work on resisting time pressure by slowing speech, by refusing to be hurried, by the use of pauses and silence is also tackled. The important message contained in this phase is that clients do not have a choice as to whether or not they stutter, but they can choose *how* they will stutter by using the above 'approach' techniques.

5 *Safety margins* are introduced to maintain a balance between the speaker's need to be fluent and the capacity to be fluent. Sheehan urges clients to 'show the other person at all times more stuttering and less perfect speech than you really can deliver' (1975, p169). In this way, the fears of stuttering are constantly being handled, providing speakers with a margin of safety. Voluntary stuttering is the main strategy employed to deal with fears of stuttering.

In addition to these five phases of therapy, **Sheehan** (1975) stresses the need for continued expansion of speaking skills, for example, by joining public speaking classes or toast-master's clubs. This maintains the 'initiative' stance encouraged earlier in therapy. He is also aware that increased fluency may present clients with problems, and that most people need psychotherapeutic help to adjust to their more fluent role. 'There are two ways to be disappointed in life. One way is never to get the things you wish for; the other way is to get them' (1975, p173). Although clients gain much from increased fluency, unexpected weaknesses may be revealed. For example, people who have postponed making friends until they are fluent may now find they do not know how to set about this task. For others, relationships built around stuttering are now thrown into a state of upheaval because of the change of role in one partner.

Sheehan's therapy is directed at the elimination of avoidance strategies. It is an aggressive approach, made bearable for clients by his profound understanding of the covert aspects of stuttering. There is no promise of fluency at the end of the painful road of throwing away the crutches of stuttering, and it is not surprising that many therapists find it easier to present clients with a fluency package such as prolonged speech. If a therapist is truly committed to Sheehan's ideas, she needs to be able to give clients the conviction that this is the only way to lay the ghosts of stuttering to rest: a worthy challenge for those who have the stomach to endure the process.

(e) A Kellian view of desensitisation

In a paper on interiorised stuttering, **Levy** (1987) subtitled desensitisation as 'reconstruing stuttering'. In fact working through Van Riper's or Sheehan's recommended approaches can be viewed as giving clients an invitation to reconstrue stuttering. Constructs about listener reactions, silence, control, eye contact, attitudes to stuttering, and so on are discussed and tested in a propositional way. Clients experiment with the different fearful aspects of stuttering and frequently find that, when they focus on the listener and not on their own reactions, stuttering may be experienced quite differently. This new information challenges the old ways of construing stuttering, and clients who are open to these ideas actually begin to reconstrue stuttering.

The idea is not that they simply change from hating stuttering to loving it, but that they find new ways of understanding it, which then provides new bases for interpersonal predictions. This can be quite alarming for some people. When you are not focusing on hating stuttering and your reactions to it, what do you focus on? Van Riper and Sheehan both give us clues. For example, **Van Riper** (1973) writes about teaching his clients to be more assertive. Viewed in a Kellian way, assertiveness is not merely a recipe for standing up for yourself, but provides a framework for construing self and others that is helpful to most people who stutter. On assertiveness training courses, clients are encouraged to make predictions about how others are feeling, so that they can decide whether or not to go ahead with confronting the person. The assertive person is a diplomat, not seeking to score points, but to increase honesty and openness in relationships. In PCT terms, clients are being helped to elaborate their role constructs upon which their predictions about self in relation to others are based. A Kellian therapist would not only teach the strategies for being more assertive, but also help the client to make personal sense of these different ways of relating to others.

Because we believe that stuttering is maintained by the efforts to stop stuttering, we are convinced that desensitisation is a crucial aspect of adult stuttering therapy. Whether or not the technique chosen for a particular client falls within the speak-more-fluently or stutter-more-fluently realms, it is still possible to incorporate some work on desensitisation into the therapy approach. We are sure that taking cognisance of the 'attitude component' of stuttering will mitigate against relapse and enable our clients to feel happier about being themselves and that fluency is less likely to be accompanied by the fear of stuttering.

(f) Experiments versus assignments

Within both the block modification and the prolonged speech approaches clients are first taught to modify their speech in the context of the therapy room, and later to transfer these skills to outside situations. In block modification therapy this gap is bridged earlier on than when fluency techniques are taught. However the approaches have in common the tendency to prescribe a series of assignments which are hierarchically organised according to their anticipated level of difficulty. Success is measured in terms of the clients' ability to put speech techniques into practice in a variety of situations.

In common with the above approaches, PCT clients also use the therapy room as a laboratory for testing predictions. However, differences occur in terms of the way experiments, as compared to assignments, are set up. The focus of change is on speech when assignments are planned. When an experiment is planned, the aim is to provide clients with testable hypotheses which, when validated, will enable them to reconstrue the situation. The broader issues pertaining to the situation are taken into account: the client is asked to predict what will happen in terms of other people's reactions, how they themselves will feel and behave and what difference these factors will make to their lives. This gets away from the idea of doing great quantities of assignments such as buying ten bus tickets fluently, making ten fluent phone calls, and so on.

Consider the different approaches in the two examples given below. Barbara is finding it difficult to slow down her speech. In the course of discussing this problem she describes herself as always in a rush: she walks quickly, talks quickly, hurries here and hurries there. She is always short of time.

■ The therapist asks her to try to vary some aspect of her behaviour other than speech on the *slow—fast* dimension. Barbara suggests that she tries walking slowly for the next week. The implications of this are elaborated: what does she predict it will feel like? How will others react? Whom will it affect the most? If she can walk slowly, how does she think this will affect her ability to slow her speech down? In this situation, the therapist has tried to take the emphasis off speech, but hopes she is teaching Barbara how to experiment, what choices she can make, and how to learn from experiments.

■ The therapist suggests that Barbara tries speaking slowly for one minute the first day, two minutes the second day, three minutes the third day, and so on.

Which approach do you feel will be the most useful?

Issues in selecting an approach

As indicated at the start of this section (*see p128*) speech therapists now seem more prepared to offer different approaches to different clients. However the criteria we are using to judge who is likely to benefit from any one approach have not been validated by research. Therefore we can only raise some of the issues involved in selecting an approach, and leave therapists to draw their own conclusions.

1 *Client variables* The following list of variables in clients may be important in selecting an approach:

   (i)   Age;

   (ii)   Gender;

   (iii)   Nature of stuttering;

   (iv)   Quality of fluency;

   (v)   Attitudes to stuttering;

   (vi)   Attitudes to fluency;

   (vii)   Amount of avoidance;

   (viii) Attitudes to previous therapy;

   (ix)   Client's needs from therapy;

   (x)   View of self;

   (xi)   Client's view of therapy and preferences for:
- the type of relationship with therapist,
- role of client,
- group/individual therapy,
- intensive/weekly therapy.

2 *Therapist variables* The following variables in the therapist are likely to influence choice of approach:

   (i)   Experience;

   (ii)   Knowledge of and attitude to different approaches;

   (iii)   Time available;

   (iv)   Style of working;

   (v)   Attitude to stuttering;

   (vi)   Ability to tolerate uncertainty;

   (vii)   Preferred way of relating to clients;

   (viii) Availability of support or supervision;

   (ix)   Counselling or psychotherapy experience;

   (x)   Beliefs about the nature of stuttering;

   (xi)   Perception of client role and therapist role.

In her survey of speech therapists' views on stuttering therapy, **Cheasman** (1987) found that, among the therapists who professed to use different approaches, the three most important criteria for selecting an approach were severity, attitude to stuttering and personality. The least important criterion was the therapist's knowledge and confidence. We can only account for this latter point in terms of the nature of the questionnaire which asked therapists to specify the criteria they used, rather than to rate supplied criteria according to their importance. Whatever the case, it seems that therapists are more willing to judge their clients than themselves.

We agree with **Murphy and Fitzsimmons** (1960) who assert that the most important single variable affecting success in stuttering therapy is *the clinician*. To lay responsibility for outcome at the client's door is to evade the necessity for acquiring expertise in stuttering therapy. Therapists have a responsibility to explore their own models of therapy and to understand why they prefer some approaches to others. We believe that a therapist is more likely to select an approach that accords with her personal view of her role as a therapist and her attitudes to stuttering. For example, a therapist who finds stuttering hard to listen to might be more inclined to use a fluency technique than block modification. While we acknowledge that everyone has views on their therapeutic role, we would like to urge therapists not to be limited by attitudes of which they are unaware. Self-exploration seems to be a necessary part of being a therapist.

Looking at variables that lie within clients, we are prepared to make a few suggestions to guide therapists in selecting an approach. We hope therapists understand that these are drawn from our experience and are not substantiated by research data. All or some of the following criteria may justify the selection of each approach.

1 *Fluency techniques such as prolonged speech*

(i)   Severity of stuttering: moderate to severe;

(ii)   S.24 score of 19 or below (**Andrews and Cutler**, 1974);

(iii)   Low avoidance of stuttering;

(iv)   Fluency is rapid and urgent with little pausing;

(v)   Client wants therapy to be disciplined and structured;

(vi)   The client is not very sensitive to stuttering;

(vii)   The client has a positive attitude to using a fluency technique.

2 *Block modification therapy*

(i)   Stuttering pattern is complex, possibly fairly stereotyped regardless of target sound;

(ii)   The client has difficulty starting—laryngeal tension;

(iii)   Fluency is fairly normal sounding;

(iv)   S.24 score of 19 or higher;

(v)   High avoidance;

(vi)   The client has negative feelings about stuttering;

(vii)   The client wants to understand why they stutter;

(viii) Poor results from a fluency approach in the past;

(ix)   The client is prepared to see stuttering as something they do;

(x)   The client may feel uncomfortable if too fluent.

3 *Avoidance-reduction therapy*

(i)   Little overt stuttering, possible only silent blocks;

(ii)   S.24 score of 19 or higher (often 24);

(iii)   The client avoids in every possible way;

(iv)   It is possible that very few know that the client stutters;

(v)   It may be the client's first attempt at therapy;

(vi)   The client understands that avoidance is the problem.

Stuttering in adults is more than a speech problem. Therefore therapy must be directed to the person and not the stuttering. We recommend most strongly that therapists incorporate speech work into a psychotherapeutic approach, such as personal construct therapy. The rationale underlying this recommendation can be supported with a brief discussion of different ways of changing.

The simplest form of change can be called 'slot movement' (**Kelly**, p938). This involves sliding clients from one end of their constructs to the other. *Figure 7.1* shows a cluster of constructs which correlated highly with each other before therapy began for a client called Sheila. The asterisks denote the poles on which she placed herself at this stage.

Figure 7.1   Constructs correlating with stuttering

*stuttering	—	fluent
*lacking confidence	—	confident
*kind and caring	—	mean and nasty

Therapy was aimed at increasing fluency through the use of prolonged speech. Her construct system at the end of the course shows some apparently sweeping changes. Instead of rating herself at the *stuttering* pole, Sheila now sees herself as *fluent*. Other changes in her system have come about, such as a move from *lacking confidence* towards *confident*. While this looks hopeful, Sheila may find some of the changes less desirable. For example, when she stuttered she saw herself as *kind and caring*. Now that she is fluent, she is forced to see herself as *mean and nasty*, because of the high positive correlation between these two constructs. When change is brought about along one construct dimension, such as changes in fluency, closely related constructs are also likely to be affected. Such a client may fail to maintain fluency because of the negative implications, and be forced to retreat along the only pathways open to her: that is, her well-worn construct slots. The change, which once seemed so dramatic, was only superficial after all.

Had Sheila been invited to elaborate her view of herself as a fluent speaker, such regression might have been averted. She might have discovered that she could maintain her preferred *kind and caring* nature and *fluency* be reorganising the relationships between her constructs. In this way she might learn that these two ways of viewing herself do not necessarily relate to each other. Now when she is *kind and caring* she cannot predict her level of fluency. The close relationship between these constructs has been changed.

The other possible way in which Sheila could be helped to change is through the formation of new constructs. For example, if she develops new ways of construing other people this will affect her behaviour in relation to them, and consequently her view of herself. New role constructs may provide more useful ways of construing others than merely in terms of their reactions to stuttering. Being able to focus on different ways of relating to others is likely to lead to an increase in fluency, because the *stuttering—fluency* construct now has little importance for Sheila.

We have argued earlier for second order change, and such change can only be brought about by reconstruction. Slot movement is an example of first order change, and precipitates clients into a roller-coaster existence of a series of inexplicable ups and downs in fluency. Our responsibility as therapists is to help clients to incorporate meaningfully the changes they make in their speech into their ways of understanding themselves and others.

Issues in selecting a regime

Apart from selecting a technique to meet the particular needs of a client, the therapist is faced with the choice of offering group or individual therapy and weekly or intensive therapy. Some of the criteria for selecting the therapy regime might be as follows:

1 *Group therapy*

(i)   The client is willing or able to see things from others' points of view and relates reasonably well to people.

(ii)   If the technique to be used is prolonged speech this is very easily taught in groups.

(iii)   Clients with more interiorised stuttering benefit from group support.

(iv)   Some aspects of block modification are usefully tackled in a group, for example, identification, variation.

2 *Individual therapy*

(i)   Client has fears of groups and/or has poor social relationships.

(ii)   The client's personal problems are extensive and need time and privacy to explore; these might include depression or relationship problems.

(iii)   If a very specific problem needs tackling, and therapy is likely to be short-term, a group may be inappropriate.

(iv)   Some aspects of block modification therapy, for example, desensitisation, are easier to handle in individual therapy.

3 *Intensive therapy*

With adequate preparation for an intensive course and planned follow-up therapy, we can recommend intensive therapy to teach the following skills:

(i)   Prolonged speech: to reach normal speaking rates more quickly.
(ii)   Block modification, but with very extensive follow-up therapy.

4 *Weekly therapy*

(i)   Avoidance-reduction therapy;
(ii)   Tackling personal problems.

Summary

This chapter has covered ways of helping clients prepare for change and utilise therapy to advantage. Ideas for facilitating speech change through the design of a series of meaningful experiments have been discussed. We recognise that these ideas may make some therapists feel anxious and uncertain, and we hope we have made a convincing case for their use. Through our own experience we feel that therapy along these lines can result in lasting change and reflects time well spent.

Growth and development of the therapist

Therapists who wish to explore their attitudes and feelings about different models of therapy should turn to the final chapter (*p189*). The tasks and questions provided do not have right or wrong answers, but are intended to be personally challenging to therapists seeking self-understanding and insight into the therapeutic process.

CHAPTER 8
THE USE OF
GROUPS IN
STUTTERING THERAPY

CHAPTER 8
THE USE OF GROUPS IN STUTTERING THERAPY

Group therapy has become an increasingly positive choice of approach in stuttering therapy. As in other disciplines, speech therapists have become aware of the power and potential usefulness of groups in the process of change. Yet what actually happens during the lifetime of a group? How do we know it is happening and how can we maximise its influence?

In order to address these issues, this chapter is divided according to the different phases of the group process. Although examples are given from stuttering therapy groups, this section is not directed specifically to the teaching of techniques within the group context. Rather, the issues involved in the planning, setting up, therapy and termination of the group are explored. These do not preclude the use of techniques which form a vital part of group speech therapy, but an assumption is made that speech techniques are more familiar to speech therapists than the techniques for enabling psychological change in the group context. In the ensuing discussion ideas are drawn from a wide variety of sources, but particular reference is made to Kelly's description of group therapy in his seminal work, *The Psychology of Personal Constructs*, (1955).

The planning phase of group therapy

(a) Selection of members

Having decided to offer group therapy, the first decision facing the therapist is the selection of members for the group. For some therapists there is virtually no choice, and membership may comprise all adults who stutter and are currently receiving speech therapy at their centre. For others, who have greater numbers on their books, the process is more complex and involves deciding who would benefit from group therapy and, of those, who would benefit from the group that is being planned. **Kelly** (1955) suggests that, in selecting people for group therapy, verbal ability is less important than the willingness of the client to perceive other people's points of view. This can be ascertained from a grid, self-characterisation or their account of previous therapy and how they function in relation to other people. A person who is highly anxious about joining a group, has poor social relationships and is very suspicious of people is unlikely to benefit from group therapy initially, although he might well do so after some individual therapy geared towards developing more useful role constructs.

Finding ways of checking whether or not a person will obstruct the group process is more difficult, but just as important. The two examples that follow illustrate a 'helpful' and an 'obstructive' group member, and demonstrate the challenge facing the therapist attempting to select wisely and carefully for her group.

Example one

Lesley was a woman who was desperate to do something about her speech. She was very wary of group therapy, not being too sure how other people would behave or what they would be like. She was concerned that she might react inappropriately to their stuttering. However, she had many open-ended ideas about the group process, such as members being able to help each other, meeting people who might understand stuttering, and not having to talk all the time. Even the fact that she anticipated that the others would not be like herself stood in her favour and implied that she would approach them more openly. She became a central person in her group, encouraging people to talk about themselves and to take risks.

Example two

Stephen was an elderly man who was very keen to join a group. He was lonely and was looking for company. He had no reservations about joining a group, having been in the army. His ideas about therapy were based on his military background: he believed that he could learn anything given enough practice. He was very talkative at his interview and held quite definite ideas about a lot of things. He seemed to enjoy humour. It was possible from his one-to-one interaction at the interview to predict that he would be an obstructive group member, because of his pre-emptive approach to people and events. He was totally certain that he was right and that others agreed with him. Yet his manner was friendly, he was positive about therapy and the chance of joining a group. Not having an alternative form of therapy to offer him, we took the risk of giving him a place in a group, hoping to help him reconstrue. We were wrong to do so without first offering him individual therapy. He pre-empted all discussions about personal differences with platitudes such as, 'We're all in the same boat'. He was unable to give feedback to others in a constructive way and ignored all feedback that they gave him. He provoked arguments and used humour at inappropriate and insensitive moments.

(b) Frequency and venue of sessions

Deciding on the times and places of meetings is the next stage in the planning process. Our experience suggests that a two-hour session is ideal for weekly therapy, giving members time to establish speech control and leaving an opportunity for a group discussion or other activity. The frequency of meetings each week will vary according to the goals of the group. Depending on the length of sessions on intensive courses, regular breaks will be needed to make each day manageable.

Finding a suitable location for group meetings can be quite difficult. The setting has an effect on the ambiance of the group and may influence the ways in which group members relate to each other. We have found that privacy is of the utmost importance; for the duration of sessions, no one should be likely to wander into the room by mistake and there should be no telephone in the group therapy room. Chairs of equal size that can be placed in a circle, but also moved easily, allow the therapist to engineer good channels of communication.

(c) Aims and objectives

Determining the purpose of the group is the next task. Choosing the aims and objectives of the group is frequently tackled in a *post hoc* way: once the therapist knows who will be in the group, she then decides its purpose. Ideally, the aims of the group should be defined before members are recruited, so that the selection criteria are made explicit. For example, the therapist may decide to run a 10-week course on desensitisation to stuttering for adults. Immediately the selection criteria become apparent:

- adults who stutter;
- people who are sensitive to stuttering;
- people who are able to work in a group;
- people who want to work on attitudes to stuttering;
- stage and previous therapy experience of members should be fairly uniform.

(d) Duration of the course of therapy

As has been alluded to above, the therapist will need to determine the duration of the course of group therapy. Again this is possible to gauge once the aims of therapy have been specified. Many therapists find it useful to contract with the group to achieve certain aims within a given time period. Although this may seem over-formalised, the advantages of entering into a contract are:

1 A more equal relationship between the therapist and group members is facilitated by both sides being aware of what the group aims are.

2 Both the group members and the therapist can become involved in evaluating whether or not those aims have been achieved at the end of the time allotted to the task.

3 Neither the therapist nor the group members are forced to commit themselves to an unworkable therapeutic relationship for any length of time. Having a contract with a built-in review procedure to see how therapy is going gives both parties a way out if any problems do arise, leaving the option of referral to another agency.

4 Having short-term goals to be achieved within a given time focuses the attention of the therapist and the group and may be conducive to task achievement. Many adults who stutter feel as if they are signing on for life when they join a group.

Any contract needs to be flexible enough to cope with changes that occur as the group grows and develops. Rigid adherence to the original contract may impede progress.

(e) Evaluation of therapy

Arising out of the idea of a therapeutic contract is the notion that therapy will have to be evaluated in some way. If possible, the means for evaluating the effectiveness of therapy should be determined before the group commences. Going back to the example above of a short course on desensitisation to stuttering, the criteria used to judge the achievements of the group might be:

1 That members are able to stutter in a greater variety of situations without reacting adversely;

2 That members are able to talk about stuttering and therapy to more people than at the start of the course;

3 That members report feeling less bothered about stuttering;

4 That stuttering ceases to be the only important criterion for judging personal effectiveness in speaking situations.

(f) Leadership

The convenor of the group will need to decide on how the group is to be led, that is, by a single therapist or with another therapist or co-worker. This decision may be influenced by the size of the group or the particular activities to be used to help the members achieve their goals. If the group is to be frequently split into subgroups, having more than one leader could be advantageous. In practice, the choice is often influenced by the availability of a suitable co-leader, and whether or not it seems possible to work together in a complementary and mutually supportive way (**Whitaker**, 1985). Sharing the running of the group is useful in that mutual supervision is virtually in-built, provided that the two co-workers can trust each other sufficiently to be open in reviewing and planning sessions. We have found it useful to lead groups jointly with ex-clients, although this is not always straightforward and requires regular discussions in both planning and evaluating sessions (**Levy and Insley**, 1987).

(g) Supervision

Supervision is an issue which will be discussed in more detail in the final chapter. However, it is worth mentioning that, because of the demanding nature of group therapy, it is advisable to organise some form of supervision for both the planning and running phases of the group. Therapists may arrange this with more experienced colleagues both within and outside our own profession. The support and challenge provided by a supervisor may enable the therapist to grow and develop in ways not possible without supervision.

The planning phase is now complete. Once the group is established and running, different skills are likely to be required to help the group achieve its aims and to deal with the dynamics of the group.

Getting started

Just because most of us live and work in groups, does not imply that we have an understanding of how groups work. **Douglas** (1978) draws an analogy between group therapy and learning the rules of a game. It is impossible to play any game successfully unless the rules are known. Likewise playing the game of 'group therapy' requires rules to structure the experience of group members. In order that members derive maximum benefit from the group, one of the tasks of the leader is to ensure that 'the rules are well and truly learned' (**Douglas**, 1978, p95).

One way of arriving at a set of rules for a group is to pose a series of questions which can then form the basis of a discussion about how members would like the group to function; for example,

■ What makes a group a good group or a bad group?

■ What role would you like to play in this group?

■ What role would you like the therapist to play in this group?

Another way is to give the group a set of rules that have previously worked well. Some examples of such rules might be:

■ Whatever is said during group sessions will be kept confidential.

■ Group members should endeavour to talk directly to each other rather than through the therapist.

■ Everyone has the right to be listened to.

■ Decision making should involve everyone in the group.

Discussing and establishing rules in the formative phase of the group sets an important process in motion, enabling members to review and reflect upon how the group is working. If members are aware of ground rules, they have a language and means for pinpointing problems and areas of satisfaction with the group. This helps to promote more equality, because knowledge of group functioning can give the group leader power over and above the power she has accrued by being the person who has seen a need, and has organised and convened the group to meet that need. The therapists' style of approach is very important in determining how the group functions. In the final chapter issues to do with therapeutic style are discussed more fully than is appropriate at this stage. Suffice it to say here that self-awareness and the ability to reflect on oneself are necessary and important characteristics of a person who wishes to run a group.

Regardless of the tasks to be tackled, the therapist brings to the group a set of 'instrumental purposes' which maintain conditions that facilitate effective work. **Whitaker** (1985, pp224–5) specifies these as being:

■ to seek to conduct the group so as to maintain a general sense of safety at a level at which members feel safe enough to stay in the group and to take personal risks;

■ to seek to avoid the irredeemable collapse of structure;

■ to work toward the establishment and maintenance of norms in the group which support it as a positive medium for help;

■ to utilise events occurring in the group for the specific benefit of members;

■ to avoid doing harm; and

■ to discern and think out how to retrieve errors.

Although significant throughout the lifespan of the group, these therapeutic aims take on a special importance in the formative stage. A group will not survive unless there is some structure and usually this is provided by the therapist. In these early stages, much of what happens can be understood in terms of each member seeking to establish a role in relation to the other people in the group. **Kelly** (1955) describes this process as 'the initiation of mutual support' and suggests that the therapist should start the group with activities that will reduce threat and vulnerability until such time as each member of the group feels accepted and supported (see below). No one is likely to be able to experiment actively until a climate of safety has been established, when members feel that others in the group are willing to try to understand them.

The established phase: the group in process

(a) Learning to see events through each other's eyes

Once each member of the group has support from someone other than the therapist, the next phase in the process can get underway. Acceptance and support convey a willingness to understand others, but now what is required is that the participants actually begin to construe each other's way of seeing events. For example, instead of John saying to Mary, 'Your feelings about your stutter seem overwhelming' (indicating acceptance) now John may say, 'It's interesting that you react with fear, guilt and shame when you stutter. That's different from me, but your past experiences with authority figures were different, so I can quite understand why you have those feelings about stuttering. I suppose every time you have to deal with your boss, these feelings are uppermost in your mind'. John has taken a step in Mary's shoes and has been able to *subsume* her construing of stuttering with authority figures.

Many of the discussions at this stage focus on clarifying comments or remarks made by members of the group. Encouraging the group to check their understanding of each other by saying what they think a person meant is useful. At first, members might feel embarrassed if they are wrong, but as they get used to speculating, they may feel more able to take risks. The therapist is in a position to provide a role model for this process by being willing to check her understanding of what is said by others. Some people find it impossible to believe that other people see things differently, and may be very threatened and resort to hostile behaviour. For example, Peter says to Sue, 'You can't tell me seriously that you don't find using the phone a problem. Everyone does. Ask anyone here.' Allowing Sue to elaborate on why she does not find the phone difficult encourages Peter to contemplate both poles of the construct and offers new alternatives which he may find difficult to absorb. It may take time before Peter can tolerate a looser style of construing.

The way in which the therapist intervenes at this stage is critical. It is often difficult to gauge just when to intervene to the advantage of the group. Many interventions are directed at a particular person, and the therapist may seem to be doing individual therapy in front of the group, which does not enhance the group process. For example, while people are struggling to define their role in the group the therapist is often faced with a client who wants to discuss a specific problem in great depth. If the issue is very interesting to the therapist, she may get involved in a long discussion with the person, excluding the rest of the group, who may not understand or be able to identify with the problem under scrutiny. There is no harm in putting the problem 'on hold' until the group are ready to join in a discussion which has bearing on the problem (**Whitaker**, 1985, p238).

Before proceeding to a discussion of the next phase, it is worth examining some of the other common errors a therapist might make in the early stages of the group's life.

- The style of leadership may be restrictive, with the therapist being too dominating or pushing members too hard too soon.

- Colluding with the group by allowing an activity to persist, even though the therapist knows from experience that it will not help, is also restrictive.

- It is possible that the therapist may find one member very irritating, and may be unintentionally hard on that person. Favouring one member above others could be equally disruptive to the group.

- On occasions an over-anxious therapist might talk too much, blocking channels of communication between members of the group.

Being aware of the possibility of making mistakes is a good way of avoiding most of them, but generally it is not possible to avoid errors altogether. The openness of the therapist and her willingness to acknowledge mistakes can be very helpful to the group (**Whitaker**, 1985, pp240–4). In the end, the only way of becoming a good group therapist is through experience and the possibility of making mistakes along the way should not deter the novice therapist.

(b) Designing and implementing experiments

The next stage involves the members of the group using their understanding of each other to design and implement experiments. These occur in the context of the group, rather than involving outside people. One way of initiating this process would be for the therapist to ask the group to review its progress in terms of how each person is feeling in the group, whether or not they are satisfied with the role the therapist is playing, whether they feel understood and listened to by the others and how they feel the group is interacting.

In stuttering groups members often raise the issue of how much each person is contributing to the group. Occasionally there are complaints about one or two people talking too much, but usually some of the more active members feel unsure about how the 'quieter' members are feeling. Other points frequently raised concern the lack of feedback from the group on speech techniques. Sometimes this criticism is directed to the therapist. Issues to do with punctuality may be raised. The group may then be asked to make suggestions as to how these problems can be resolved. We usually encourage quantity of ideas at first, so that the group or group member can choose from a selection of strategies. As part of initiating these sorts of experiments in the group, it is useful to specify how validational evidence can be collected. For example, if one person is scared of criticising another's speech, we might ask the group to say 'thank you' when that member gives feedback, and later discuss what it felt like for him to give feedback.

This phase of the group process enables the original ground rules to become group norms. Ground rules cannot be enforced without consent from the group. Having a ground rule such as 'Everyone will give and receive feedback' will only become an established norm when the members have experience of both giving and receiving feedback. By creating experiments for each other and being willing to test out hypotheses, the participants are also learning about the process of change. So far their experiments are confined to the context of the group, but the methodology of experimenting in a manageable and structured way is being learned.

By this stage, the group will have dealt with some of the conflicts between members and have an established way of working. Trust and support are likely to have been extended, and members will feel safe enough to begin to explore problems in greater depth and to find solutions emerging from group discussions. As long as the group is moving towards its goals, the group therapist can take a back seat, only intervening to redirect the group to the task it has set for itself. Earlier on the group leader will have needed to be more active, since the group were less aware of what needed to be done, but by now they will have learned how to work in a group and require less direction from the therapist.

The role of the therapist during this established phase of the group process is of great importance. One of the objectives of group therapy is that clients learn to disperse their dependencies. If the therapist is very directive and controlling, the group members will become over-dependent on her and progress will be hampered. Group therapy also aims to demonstrate to people just how capable they are of solving problems. By encouraging participants to put forward their ideas, which may be taken up by the person whose problem is under discussion, individuals begin to discover their own potential for problem solving. This increases their autonomy in the long term, because they will have gained insight into the problem-solving process. Again, if the therapist is too eager to demonstrate her skill and expertise in finding solutions, members may feel helpless and dependent and the whole point of group therapy will have been lost.

(c) Exploration of personal problems

The established phase of group therapy is geared towards personal change. Problems may be raised and discussed in detail by the group. *Enactment* is a useful technique for demonstrating what went wrong in a particular situation outside therapy. The other members may like to try and enact the situation, showing how they might deal with the problem, in this way presenting the person with alternative ways of viewing the situation. In the discussion following the enactments, constructs can be elicited and thus made explicit.

For example, Sam says that people are always laughing at him when he says goodbye at work. When he enacts the situation, the group becomes aware of how he shuffles through the door and seems apologetic. Others enact the situation differently, focusing on different body language—eye contact, posture, speed of walking. When we discuss the enactment afterwards, it emerges that for Sam leaving work arouses tremendous guilt. He feels he is being evaluated on one of his core constructs: *lazy-hardworking*. Any remark from colleagues which seems to place him on the *lazy* pole dislodges him from his core role. The group help him to construe the situation differently by asking him to take on the parts of colleagues who taunt him as he leaves work. He then realises that they are teasing him and are validating his hardworking nature, rather than criticising him. Next he reverses roles, taking on his own part and tries to walk through the door in a more matter-of-fact way, focusing on the prediction that teasing is friendly and that he can answer back. In response to, 'Going home so early!' he manages to say, 'Got to leave something for tomorrow'. This enactment leads on to a commitment from Sam to experiment during the week.

What has happened here is important for Sam. His original construction of the situation had to do with how he construed himself. By the time the group had completed the enactment and discussed the situation he was able to use role constructs which focused on his relationship with his colleagues, and now the situation became one of exchanging 'strokes' rather than a test of his worth as a worker. This reconstruction freed him to elaborate other constructs about himself in relation to others.

Discussions about problems are another useful activity at this stage. The kinds of issues raised will depend very much on the overall aims of the group. Because we view stuttering as affecting the whole person, we are inclined not to impose limits on the type of subjects people wish to discuss. What is important is that the whole group can respond to the discussion, and that the session does not degenerate into a dialogue.

For example, in an evening class it became apparent during the review of the week that everyone was grappling with problems to do with work. Some people wanted to change jobs, others were unemployed, another wanted to change careers and one person was debating whether or not to seek employment for the first time. In the ensuing discussion the therapist noted that the group were reassuring rather than challenging each other and that the discussion was going round in circles. One person even said that the group was in this very mess because they were coming to speech therapy!

The therapist intervened to provide the group with a focus. She suggested that each person try to say what they were finding threatening about the thought of changing their employment status. This led to a very different discussion. There was commonality in terms of the theme, but highly individual reactions to change. Joe was a solicitor and wanted to give up law. His threats had to do with his family's reactions to this after so many years invested in law. Mary was bored with her job, but found the thought of the unknown, or learning new things, very threatening. Josie felt that her role as mother and wife was under threat if she went out and looked for work, and so on. We then proceeded to discuss strategies for dealing with threat in general and each person's threat in particular. By the end of the evening everyone left with a manageable task to pursue in the week. Joe was asked to write down all the factors influencing his decision and to put these in order of priority. Mary agreed to ask someone at work to show her how to use the word processor, so that she could look at how she found learning a new task. Josie was asked to draw up a timetable for her week to find out how many hours she had free after being a sufficiently good mother and wife to her own satisfaction.

There is another interesting twist to this tale. The therapist was also involved in changing jobs at this point and decided to discuss her own threats, which involved a change in role relationships. She too was given a task, which was to discuss the implications of the new job with one colleague in order to discover how this person viewed the impending change. Needless to say, much was gained from the venture! The group seemed pleased to have been of help and the experience was very validating for all concerned.

(d) Construing outsiders' points of view

As people become more able to take risks in the group, so their behaviour outside therapy begins to change. Clients may begin to interpret the points of view of people they know outside. The therapist needs to ensure that the group members are making a real effort to subsume the outlook of these other persons, and that they are not merely seeking to validate their own constructions.

An example springs to mind of a client, Rob, who was very insistent that we 'cure' him. When speaking of interviews or encounters with others he evaluated his performance entirely on the basis of how tolerant listeners were to his stuttering. He insisted that no future employer could possibly have time to be tolerant. As the kinds of jobs he was seeking involved computing, we were puzzled by the high priority he placed on fluency for work. At interviews he had had some feedback that his speech was not a criterion for judging his fitness for the job. He could not or would not believe this. When others in the group from fairly high-powered computing jobs said that their speech did not affect their career prospects, he discounted their comments. He was unable to use the neutral reactions of speech therapists or other people who stuttered or even his friends to alter his perspective.

We could not find out why he was holding on to this very pre-emptive view of people, until he mentioned in passing that when he was quite young his mother had said that she found his stuttering irritating. For him this implied that *he* was irritating, and this was the prediction he tested every time he opened his mouth to speak. This over-used construct provided him with the only meaningful way of relating to others. People divided neatly into two categories: those who found him irritating and those who could tolerate his stutter. It was no wonder that fluency was the only solution to his predicament that he could find. Any alternative was very threatening and meaningless. His attempt to interpret the points of view of others was hostile in the sense that he was extorting evidence to support his theory, and not making a speculative guess at how others might view things.

Because he had made such a major investment in this construct it was highly resistant to change and, certainly on the intensive course, we found no way of helping him to surrender his pre-emptive way of construing.

(e) Generalisation of role constructs

Kelly (1955) suggests that this stage can be used to generalise the role constructs members have developed in the group to people outside. Through discussion of the similarities or differences between people inside and outside the group, the permeability of their role constructs is likely to be increased. Instead of a construct now being relevant only to group members, it becomes useful for making predictions about people in general. Once group members discover that they can relate meaningfully to people outside the group, they are likely to feel less dependent on the therapy situation as the only place where they feel understood or where they can understand others. The process of role construing has been set in motion, and the person is free to experiment with and elaborate his view of others.

Therapists will recognise that this phase has begun when the content of group discussions begins to change. There will be more talk of outside ventures and less talk of particularly painful situations. For example, Lesley suddenly told her group that she had joined a public speaking class, and that she had told them that she stuttered and had received support and admiration from them. She told her speech therapy group that she would come to therapy every second week only, if that was all right with them, as the public speaking class required a lot of work and time. She had been able to generalise constructs about listener reactions to stuttering from her therapy group to the public speaking class, and found that they were useful predictors of others' behaviour. The validational evidence thus collected made her therapy group less distinctive as the only forum where she could discuss stuttering. Lesley was actively elaborating role constructs and experimenting with change.

Throughout this discussion of the three main activities comprising the established phase of group therapy, that is, enactment, discussions about personal problems and the elaboration and generalisation of role constructs, emphasis has been placed on experimenting with change. This has been discussed more fully in previous chapters. We would like to stress here how important it is to encourage active experimentation both inside and outside the group, while keeping threat and anxiety manageable. Experimentation has several functions which are essential to ultimate change.

■ Firstly, it provides the client with a framework of anticipation: a way of predicting the outcome of behavioural change.

■ Secondly, instead of therapy being mere speculation and intellectualisation, the client is brought into contact with reality.

■ Thirdly, experimentation enables the client to test his construct system.

■ Fourthly, the therapist is given the chance to evaluate therapy and to see how adequately she has construed the client's situation.

■ Fifthly, active experimentation opens up new vistas of experience, as was illustrated in the example of Lesley above.

■ Finally, the client gets to make contact with other people and to learn how others see the world. In order to do this successfully, role constructs will need to be developed and tested (**Kelly**, 1955, pp1125–7).

Terminating and evaluating therapy

'Terminating means finishing, stopping, separating, leaving', (**Whitaker**, 1985, p363). Because of the implications of loss and separation, it is important that the termination phase be seen as an integral part of the total group process: as a symbol of growth rather than loss (**Douglas**, 1976).

During the planning phase, the therapist will have made some estimation of the duration of the group. With a closed group this tends to imply that therapy will end for all members at the same time. With an open group, some members will leave to be replaced by others. Their leaving is no less important than when the group closes down as a whole, and the same kind of planning and care needs to be taken for both endings. Shorter groups that run for 10–12 sessions may require less time devoted to termination than a longer-term group. The more intensive therapy has been, the more structured the closing phases will need to be (**Douglas**, 1976). Whatever the case, members need to be notified that the group is drawing to a close. Very often acknowledgement of this fact influences the manner in which members participate in the final stages of therapy. Issues to do with anticipating the separation, self assessment and planning for the future merit discussion and, therefore, devoting a specified period to termination is indicated.

As in the early stages of group life, the therapist takes responsibility for winding down the group. In effect this involves the reverse process of getting the group going in the first instance. Now ties within the group need to be slackened, while ties outside the group are strengthened (**Douglas**, 1978). The group needs time to anticipate the ways in which they will manage without the group structure. Talking about the things they might miss or things they will not miss helps to clarify these feelings (**Whitaker**, 1985). Allowing for sentimentality enables members to deal with their feelings and may prevent the huge let-down after the final session. Often the therapist or some members of the group feel embarrassed by the emotional content of discussions at the leaving stage, and may block such talk with reassuring comments such as 'Don't worry, you'll be fine'.

Although **Kelly** (1955) does not specifically discuss terminating therapy, there are two points which he raises that are applicable to this stage. The first has already been mentioned and concerns the dispersal of dependencies. Group therapy, as opposed to individual therapy, facilitates this process by virtue of the numbers of people involved in the therapeutic process. In the final stages of therapy the client will be engaging in enterprises outside the therapeutic arena and should be encouraged to continue to do so. Kelly cautions therapists not to become jealous as clients demonstrate their decreasing dependency on both the therapist and the group.

The second point involves the tightening of constructs to provide the client with an anticipatory structure for the future. This can be done by asking the group to reflect on itself, drawing out constructs to do with dependency and change. It can also take the form of summarising or stock-taking. Members of the group can be encouraged to write reports on themselves, an activity which serves to tighten up and make accessible the chief construct dimensions along which they have moved. Members might be asked to comment on each other's progress, which provides alternative constructions. It is interesting how often changes made by a person are trivialised by himself, and yet thought to be significant moves by others in the group. These discussions can give all members a broader way of viewing change, and validational evidence can be collected from a group used to giving feedback.

In the planning phase it was suggested that, if the therapist specified the aims of the group, criteria for evaluating whether or not those goals had been achieved would be apparent. It might be useful to the group if these points are raised and the therapist provides the group with feedback as to how they have progressed. A word of caution, though: if the group has not been successful in attaining their objectives, this process might be destructive and therefore contra-indicated. In such a case, this might be a task to be taken up between the therapist and her supervisor.

Evaluation of therapy in some form or other is necessary in order to plan for future therapy. Even though the life of the group is over, the process of change or need for help might not be over for some or all members of the group. In some cases, renegotiation of the original contract might be appropriate, extending the life of the group. In other cases, referral of members who need more help for individual therapy or to another group is indicated.

Finally, the group may decide on a ritualistic ending to their group such as going out for a drink or making farewell speeches. These rituals serve the function of helping the participants to take their leave from the group and give everyone a sense that it is right that the group has come to an end (**Whitaker**, 1985).

Group activities

In the section below we have included some of the activities and exercises that we have found useful with groups of people who stutter. They are drawn from many sources: from our own experience, books and from colleagues and clients. We hope that our ideas will stimulate therapists to create their own material. While we have attempted to group the exercises according to the different phases of the therapy process, we leave therapists with the responsibility for using the activities at the appropriate times and for making the connection between the activity and their overall therapy aims.

In the final chapter we have included a series of tasks which therapists might find useful to tackle prior to starting a group. We strongly recommend that therapists work through these before using the activities outlined below. An increased awareness of what is involved will enable therapists to select activities more appropriately and enhance their contribution following an activity.

(a) Criteria for selecting a group activity

The following list is intended to help therapists evaluate a particular activity against the needs of the group at any stage of therapy:

1 The current aims of the group:
   ■ Speech: have the group enough control over stuttering to meet the communicative demands of the exercise?
   ■ Group process: what stage has the group reached and what is required to help them move on?
   ■ Does the activity correspond to the specific aims of the group?
2 Is the amount of anxiety involved manageable?
3 The verbal ability of the group:

   ■ age,
   ■ educational background,
   ■ interests.
4 Is the exercise structured/unstructured?
   Which is more useful to the group now?

5 How much time is required for the activity?

6 How many people are needed for the exercise?

7 What will the group gain from the exercise?

(b) Getting to know each other

(i) Who am I? (15 mins)

At the start of a stuttering therapy group, no one is particularly keen to speak. It is helpful if the group members can get to know something about each other. One way is via this useful activity from *Gamesters' Handbook* (**Brandes and Phillips**, 1978).

- Everyone writes 10 things about themselves, including their names, on a piece of paper;
- Pin or stick the pieces of paper to their chests;
- Instruct the group to mill around until they have read each person's list.

(ii) Line-ups (5 mins)

Line-ups can be used to portray the deeper relationships within groups, but we have adapted this exercise for use in the 'getting to know each other' stage. The aim is to create a situation where everyone has to interact and move around. All or any of the following may be used.

- Ask the group to arrange themselves in a line alphabetically;
- Ask the group to arrange themselves according to who travelled the furthest to get to therapy;
- According to who has had the biggest breakfast;
- According to age;
- According to height; and so on.

(iii) Name games (10 mins)

Sitting in a circle, each person is asked to think of an adjective that begins with the same sound as their name. Then the first person introduces herself, for example:

Serious Celia (alliteration wins out!).

The next person repeats the first adjective and name and then adds their own;

Serious Celia,
Reflective Rosemarie;

and so on, until everyone has been included. It may be appropriate to ask the group to spot any themes in the adjectives.

(iv) Encouraging the use of names

Because of the difficulty of saying words which cannot be avoided and also because of the general level of anxiety in groups, people who stammer very seldom use each other's names during discussions. Early on in the life of a group the therapist can suggest that everyone uses a person's name when they are addressing a comment directly to that person. Three important gains are made from so doing:

- the speaker is more likely to be listened to;
- socially it is appropriate to use people's names and therefore this skill is transferable to outside;

- using people's names tackles the general problem of avoidance.

(c) Warm-up exercises

These exercises are for use at the start of any session at any stage of the course of therapy. Their function is to loosen up the group and to get people interacting more freely with each other.

(i) The human knot (10 mins)

Ask the group to stand shoulder to shoulder and stretch out their arms in front of them. With eyes shut, each person grabs hold of any two hands they can find. The task is to untangle the knot and end up in a circle without letting go hands.

(ii) A kind of musical chairs (10 mins)

One person stands in the middle of the group, who are seated in a circle around him. There are no vacant chairs. The person in the middle gives an instruction such as, 'Everyone wearing something blue, change seats', and when they do, he tries to get himself a seat. One person will not have a seat and has to continue to find issues relevant to those present to get as many people as possible to change seats; for example: 'All those who voted Labour, change seats', 'All those who are happy, change seats', 'All those who watch Dallas, change seats'. The game has no end of its own, and the therapist may call 'time' at the appropriate point.

(iii) The good news and the bad news (10 mins)

This idea comes from the BBC radio programme, *I'm sorry I haven't a clue* and is suitable for a fairly humorous and articulate group. One person starts off a story with 'the good news', the next person counters with 'the bad news', and, going round the circle, the next person states 'the good news', and so on until the story dies. For example, 'The good news is, we're going on a cruise'; 'The bad news is, it's a cruise missile'; 'The good news is, I've always wanted to visit Moscow'; 'The bad news is, this one's going to Washington', and so on.

(d) Activities to promote support and acceptance

(i) Why are you here? (30 mins)

This is by nature more of a discussion than a game. The group is not expected to show understanding yet, but rather a willingness to listen to and accept what each member is saying. The time has come when it is appropriate for members to share their aims and objectives for the course with each other. We ask the group to write down three personal aims for themselves which are then discussed (**Reid**, 1987).

(ii) Theories about stuttering (30 mins)

Again this activity takes the form of a discussion. The group members are asked to elaborate on their theories about stuttering. Questions such as those being used by Carolyn Cheasman in her research might be useful prompts:

- What sort of problem do you think stuttering is?
- Do you think you can liken it to any other problem? If not, why not?
- What do you think causes stuttering?
- What do you think keeps your stuttering going?

- Does stuttering vary according to the situation—why do you think this is so?
- Do you think you'd be a different sort of person if you didn't stutter?

(iii) Words to describe stuttering and fluency (30 mins)

A common language is needed to help the group to identify the overt features of their speech. Collecting the words each person uses to describe the different types of stuttering, and asking people to demonstrate what they mean, helps the group to broaden its view of stuttering. Having words to describe fluency is also useful and, if it is broken down into a series of skills, fluency loses some of its mystery. During this exercise we ask the group not to describe their feelings or reactions to stuttering, but rather its visible and observable aspects. Some useful words are:

Stuttering		Fluency
block	repetition	rate of speech
prolongation	hesitation	intonation
tension	avoidance	rhythm
eye contact	facial movements	flow
hand movements	backtracking	volume
fillers	starters	pausing

(e) Exercises to encourage trust and increase safety

(i) Obstacle course (20–30 mins)

One person is asked to leave the room. The rest of the group rearrange the furniture as an obstacle course, and stand round the edge of the room. Then the person outside is asked to shut her eyes and is led into the room by one of the members. She is then talked through the obstacle course by the group, who each take a turn at guiding the person through a part of it. If the person becomes frightened at any point, she may open her eyes or ask for help. Apart from being led in, there is no touching involved in this exercise which relies solely on promoting safety through the tone of the voice.

The obstacle course can be altered and other people may volunteer to be talked through it.

(ii) What's in a name? (30–45 mins)

This activity involves revealing personal information, but each person is in charge of how far to take their contribution. The group members are asked to tell the story behind how they got their name. Further questions may include:

- What would you like to have been called?
- If you had been of the opposite sex what would you have been called?
- What nicknames have you had over the years?
- If you did not stutter, would you need a new name?

(f) Exercises to promote group cohesion

(i) *Generating group norms (30 mins)*

This useful exercise is adapted from **Johnson and Johnson** (1982). The group is split into subgroups of twos and threes and each small group is asked to list five 'do's and five 'don'ts' for group members. When the groups join up, they are asked to share their lists. Finally, the whole group is asked to agree on three 'do's' and 'don'ts' which affect group cohesion the most.

(ii) *Evaluation discussion (20 mins)*

Even though the group seems to have agreed rules or norms to govern the way in which members work together, it is useful to review group functioning periodically. On intensive courses we do this each week: on evening classes, every six weeks or so. The following check list (**Douglas**, 1976) can be used as the basis of such a discussion, or may be useful for evaluating how a group tackled a particular exercise. Each person is given their own copy.

1. What was the general atmosphere in the group?	
Formal	Informal
Competitive	Co-operative
Hostile	Supportive
Inhibited	Permissive
COMMENTS	

2. Quantity and quality of work accomplished		
Accomplishment:	High	Low
Quality of Production:	High	Low
Goals:	Clear	Vague
Methods:	Clear	Vague
COMMENTS		

3. Leadership behaviour	
Attentive to group needs	Dominated group
Supported others	Took sides
Concerned with only one topic	Helped group
COMMENTS	

4. Participation	
Most people talked	Only a few talked
Members involved	Members apathetic
Group united	Group divided
COMMENTS	

(g) Activities to encourage subsuming

Group cohesion will also be influenced by the extent to which members can understand and see things from each others' point of view.

(i) Group iceberg (45 minutes)

Sheehan (1958) drew the well-known analogy between stuttering and an iceberg. In both, only the tip shows, while the greater part lurks below the surface. This activity aims to draw out the hidden component of stuttering, which usually comprises feelings, memories of speaking failure, reactions to stuttering and the certain knowledge that the problem will not just disappear. The therapist draws an 'iceberg' on a board or flipchart and calls on the members of the group to name those feelings and reactions experienced before, during and after stuttering. As people offer contributions, the therapist fills these into the lower part of the iceberg. More importantly, when the group is asked who feels similarly, the potential for supporting and understanding each other is increased. Many of the feelings and memories of painful experiences linked with stuttering are likely to be shared and understood by others who stutter. Talking about these feelings and memories may be very cathartic for the group.

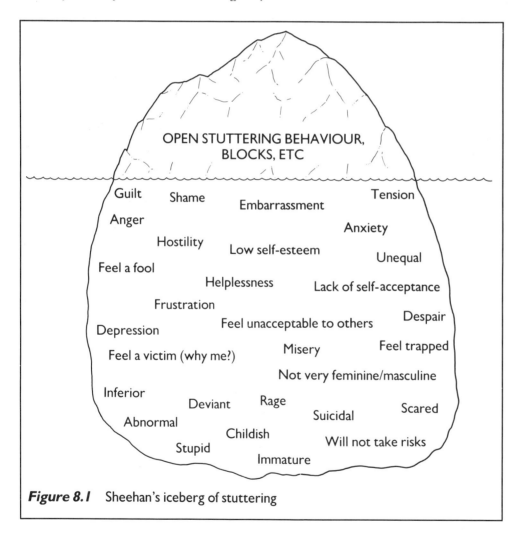

Figure 8.1 Sheehan's iceberg of stuttering

(ii) Identifying the overt features of stuttering (2–4 hours)

Armed with their vocabulary of words to describe stuttering and fluency, the group can be split into pairs and set the task of describing all they can see and hear each other do during speaking. The group needs to be directed to use descriptive rather than evaluative language. They can be asked to observe and report back to each other on instances of each of the following behaviours:

- fluent utterances;
- easy stutters;
- avoidance behaviours;
- core stuttering behaviours.

Having done this, they are asked to imitate aspects of each other's stuttering behaviour. This task involves the ability to construe stuttering non-verbally and, if accurately done, gives the imitator an insight into his partner's experiences of stuttering. **Van Riper** (1973) stresses the importance of the therapist being able to 'get his client's stuttering into his own mouth', and therefore therapist involvement in this exercise is useful.

(iii) *Matching feelings to aspects of stuttering (30 mins)*

This task completes identification and provides each group member with a fairly comprehensive appreciation of what it is like to stutter the way others in the group do. The words, 'I observe' and 'therefore I imagine' are central to this exercise. Each person is asked to make an observation about some aspect of another person's speech, and then to state what they imagine the person feels like when they speak that way. The group is split into pairs again. Person A is asked to speak while person B observes. Then person B gives feedback in the following way: '*I observe* you purse up your lips and push to get the word out. *I imagine* you feel as if the word will never come out. Maybe a bit panicky'.

Person A then confirms or elaborates on her feelings, and they continue until most features of A's stuttering have been linked to feelings from the iceberg. Then they exchange tasks.

(iv) *Presentation of a self characterisation (2 hours minimum)*

This task has been adapted by **Levy** (1987) from Kelly's way of using the self characterisation. Each person in the group is asked to talk about themselves in the third person, painting as full a picture as is possible. The rest of the group is asked to listen credulously, to believe that what each person says is true for them. After each presentation the group may ask questions, preserving the use of the third person to maintain the slight distance and protection that this affords.

For example, if Richard has said, 'Richard is the sort of person who believes his stutter is the most important thing about him' a question may follow, such as 'Why does Richard think stuttering is so important?' Richard may answer, 'Because it is all Richard thinks about, no matter what he is doing or where he is. It is always there'.

Once the group has finished exploring Richard's view of himself, they can proceed to the next person. On one of our evening classes we found it useful to tackle one character sketch each week.

(h) Tasks highlighting communication within groups

The purpose of such tasks is to highlight the way in which information is communicated in the group during problem solving, and may lead on to designing experiments to change patterns of behaviour. Although the full exercises will not be described here, the procedures for incorporating them into group therapy will. The two examples are drawn from two editions of the same book, *Joining Together* by **Johnson and Johnson** (1975, 1982) and are called 'The Murder Mystery' and the 'Solstice-Shenanigans Mystery'. Although the content is different, the procedures are identical.

These exercises involve each member of the group being given cards which contain clues to solve the mysteries. The group is asked not to show their cards to each other. Then they are told that as a group they have enough information between them to solve the mystery. They are not in competition with each other, but rather are required to reach consensus within 30 minutes as to who perpetrated the crime, when, why and how. We usually say that as therapists we will not participate in the exercise, and that after they get started we will not answer any further questions. The only other instruction we give groups is that they may not write, but otherwise they are free to solve the mystery by whatever means they choose.

Usually groups are very lost at the start, and look to the therapist for guidance. We have found it more useful not to help them than to be tempted to make suggestions. After a while they do get going and people are able to develop different roles in the process of solving the mystery.

Johnson and Johnson (1982, p195) suggest that the following analysis of group communication be made after the mystery is solved:

1 What were the patterns of communication in the group? Who spoke? To whom? How often? For how long? What could have been done to gain wider participation?

2 Was information easily obtained by all members of the group? Did all people share information appropriately?

3 Were the resources of all group members used? Was everyone listened to?

4 How did the group make decisions?

5 What problems did the group have in working together?

6 What conclusions about communication can be made from the group's experience?

(i) Designing and implementing experiments in the group

The tasks described in the previous section may identify problems in terms of the ways in which the group communicates. In order to find alternative strategies, the following exercises may be used:

(i) Finding alternative predictions

Ask each person to write down a short phrase to describe the sort of role they would like to play in the group. Then ask them to say what the opposite of that role might be. For example, Elizabeth would like to be constructive as opposed to being destructive and over-critical.

The next question for the group is, 'How might such a person feel?' Elizabeth thinks that a constructive person would probably feel *quietly confident,* while a destructive person would *always want to score points off others.*

The next question is, 'How might such a person behave?' Elizabeth tells us that a constructive person would *give positive and negative feedback that took account of how others might be feeling* whereas someone who was destructive and over-critical would *only give negative feedback.*

Finally, having elaborated a possible new role, Elizabeth might be asked to give examples of constructive criticism and to see if she felt quietly confident. The group is invited to give feedback, until such time as Elizabeth feels she has modified her behaviour to her satisfaction.

The important point in this approach is that we did not need to know much about how Elizabeth saw her role before she began to change it. Maybe

162

she felt she was over-critical, maybe too talkative? It really does not matter. This method of elaborating the feeling and behavioural components of constructs is attributable to **Leitner** (1981).

(ii) Variations

To encourage experimentation generally and to enable the group to take a more serious look at the implications of change, we have used Van Riper's suggestion that people be encouraged to vary aspects of their non-speech behaviour. Rather than trying to improve themselves, the idea here is that people tackle doing something different in the hope that they may learn about the process of change. At the appropriate point in therapy, the group is asked to think of tasks each member could tackle outside the group. The criteria for selecting such a task are:

1 That it results in noticeable change;
2 That it is small enough to be manageable;
3 That it involves the person in changing something quite important to them; and, incidentally,
4 That they do not tell anyone why they are doing it.

The group is urged to approach this playfully, but thoughtfully. These experiments need to be based on an understanding by the group of what each person is like. Once everyone, including the therapist, has their instructions, each person may be asked to make predictions about other people's reactions. They may also be asked how they will feel doing the task. Some examples of changes that group members have tackled include:

■ buying a different newspaper,
■ shaving off a moustache,
■ changing a hairstyle.

The change need not be momentous to be important to the person involved. Some groups find this exercise very useful and seem to get a lot out of the discussions about change.

(j) Discussions

During the process of group therapy with people who stutter there are many topics that are worth discussing. The list that follows includes some which we have found useful. They are not ordered in any meaningful way. Therapists are left to make their own choice as to which topics to follow up.

When holding a group discussion, it is not always easy to involve everyone. The more articulate members may dominate the discussion, leaving the less articulate members feeling inadequate or bored. We have found it useful to prepare the ground for discussions by breaking the group into subgroups of twos or threes, with specific questions to answer in relation to the chosen topic. These questions invite group members to relate the topic to themselves by asking for examples from their own lives. Once everyone is involved in the topic, but has not run out of steam, we bring the group together to share what they have discussed so far and expand where possible. Asking a group member to chair the discussion gives the group a new experience and frees the therapist to observe the group process.

For example, take our first topic for discussion: Change. In pairs, members can discuss the following sub-questions:

■ Why might change be easy or difficult for you?

- If you were to change in some important way, what would the consequences be—for yourself and for others?

Questions like these get group members thinking and provide the group with many personal examples when brought together to discuss further issues to do with change.

List of possible topics:

- Change; the threats and anxieties of change;
- Fears of fluency;
- Assertiveness;
- Strategies for dealing with stress;
- Strategies for dealing with unexpected stuttering;
- Making choices: knowing what is best for yourself;
- Taking risks;
- Past events that have influenced the rest of your life;
- Keeping motivated to work on speech;
- Evaluating your own progress;
- Body language;
- Becoming a more fluent person: catching up on lost experience;
- Conversation;
- Getting to know people;
- Job interviews;
- Learning to listen;
- What to tell people about stuttering and therapy;
- Relapse;
- Relaxation;
- Decreasing avoidance;
- Finding out how others see you;
- The telephone;
- What do fluent people think about?
- Tolerating variability in speech.

(k) Enactment to promote role construing

The following exercises make use of Kelly's technique of enactment, described more fully above and in *chapter three*. The aim of these enactments is to assess the usefulness of constructs to do with relating to other people.

(i) *Spontaneous elaboration*

A situation is created which will involve all members of the group. Each person is given a card which tells them who they are and a little bit about what they are like. The role need not be designed to 'improve' the social behaviour of people in the group, but rather to give them permission to use a different approach. For example, the card might say, 'You are a police officer, but try hard to forget this when you're not in uniform, as now'. Members are asked not to show their cards to each other, but to think about how the words on their card will affect their behaviour. Then the group is warned that they may not make any assumptions about each other based on past knowledge. To all intents and purposes they have just met, and have to find out who they think they will get along with best. The scene could be a cocktail party. The group is given 10 to 15 minutes to form first impressions of the people present.

Later they can discuss how they found out important things about each other, why they liked certain people, why they did not like others. What were their first impressions? How did they make predictions about each other? Because each person is protected by the role they were asked to play, the discussion can be more open than if they were talking about their 'real' selves.

(ii) Corners

The group are divided into three or four subgroups of two to three people each. Each subgroup is assigned to a corner of the room. Each corner is given a name: Parents' Corner, Siblings' Corner, Teachers' Corner, Friends' Corner. When people are in a particular corner they are asked to take on the role of one of their parents, siblings, teachers or friends. They are asked to talk about themselves as they were at a particular age, say six years old, but through the eyes of whichever associate they happen to be.

For example, Mary takes on the role of her mother and discusses Mary at six years old with one of the other 'parents' in the Parents' Corner. Every 10 minutes people are asked to change corners until everyone has been in all the corners relevant for them.

The debriefing discussion afterwards can focus on historical constructs that have influenced people's lives. Very often group members gain insight into how their parents felt around the time when they had just started or were developing stuttering. For those who find it hard to forgive their parents, teachers, friends or siblings, seeing events through other eyes can be useful.

There are many variations to this exercise. The whole group could be asked to be parents of children who stammer and to discuss their feelings and concerns. The group could be asked to be their own colleagues from work, and discuss what it is like to work with someone who stutters. At the end the group is not asked to like or sympathise with these other people, simply to explore alternative constructions of events. The important issue is that they are given the opportunity to see things through other people's eyes, which may help them elaborate their understanding of these outside people. This activity has been adapted from **Kelly** (1955).

(iii) 'Scruples'

This game is commercially available and provides a wonderful opportunity for validating predictions about what people might do in various problem situations. A member of the group selects one person in the group and reads one of the 'dilemma' cards to that person, who has to reply 'Yes', 'No', or 'Depends'. The group may challenge the answer if they believe the person is lying and in the end the group votes as to whether or not they believe what has been said. The game involves putting constructs on the line for testing!

Because the dilemmas tend to be rather amusing, playing 'Scruples' can be good fun as well as serving useful therapeutic purposes.

(l) Exercises to promote the generalisation of role constructs

Following on from the enactment in the previous section, group members may be asked to test some of the constructs they found useful in forming first impressions. How they do this needs to be planned and discussed.

For example, Harry found some people *more responsive* during the 'cocktail party' enactment. When we explored this further, looking at what behaviours in Harry had elicited responsive behaviours in his listeners, we discovered that his eye contact had been good, and that he had given good listening signals such as nodding and 'uhuh'- type noises of encouragement. On the basis of this, Harry was asked to put some of these behaviours into action with another person outside therapy, whom he predicted would be responsive. The group decided with Harry that responsive behaviour involved saying more than 'yes' or 'no' to questions. He had been set an experiment to test the validity of a role construct formed in the therapy room in an outside situation.

Another way of enabling members to generalise role constructs might be to ask the group to write down on a small piece of paper one thing that they admire about anyone in the group. They are also asked to give its opposite. The context must have something to do with the way the admired person relates to others, for example, *smiles warmly—solemn*. The pieces of paper are folded and placed in the middle of the room. Each person picks one, and commits themselves to using this construct in an experiment during the week. If the construct they pick is way outside the range of convenience of their system, they may have another choice. Borrowing other people's constructs is not always ideal, but may free a person to conduct a novel experiment.

(m) Terminating therapy

As the life of a group draws to a close, there are a few tasks that help members take their leave of the group.

(i) Discussion topics

1 Is there anything that needs to be resolved, discussed, dealt with or expressed before the group ends? (**Johnson and Johnson**, 1982, p462).
2 The important experiences in the group.
3 Things I will miss.
4 Things I won't miss.
5 What it's been like being a member of this group.

(ii) Report writing

Before the last session, each person can be asked to write a report evaluating their progress. We have found the following headings to be useful:

1 Progress made on the course.
2 Attitudes to speech and therapy.
3 Role in the group.
4 Factors affecting future progress.

(iii) Parting gifts

Pin a blank piece of paper to each person's back. Everyone writes something positive about that person on their sheet of paper. An alternative way is that people express their feedback verbally.

(iv) Group photograph

Without discussing it, the group is asked to get into position for a group photograph. Each person in turn steps out of the 'picture' and looks at the group. If they want to make changes to the positions or expressions on anyone's faces they may do so until they get the 'picture' they want to remember.

(v) Toasting

Each person in turn proposes a toast to the group as they leave.

(vi) Group hug

The group huddle close together in a circle, with arms round the outside and gives itself a hug.

(vii) And finally . . .

Johnson and Johnson (1982) suggest that each member of the group writes a contract with themselves to make some changes in their lives. It may involve starting something new, stopping something old, or changing some current aspect of life. It should involve generalising some of the skills acquired in the group to life outside the group. The contracts can be left in stamped, addressed envelopes with the therapist to be posted to members three months after the course finishes.

CHAPTER 9
CONTINUING
THE PROCESS
OF CHANGE

CHAPTER 9
CONTINUING
THE PROCESS
OF CHANGE

This chapter is concerned with two issues which are interrelated: first, a theory of relapse, for we believe that if therapists understand more about why their clients may regress, they may be able to prevent it; and second, ways of helping clients to continue to change their views of themselves and others after they have tackled direct work on speech. In many stuttering texts, a chapter such as this would be entitled 'The Maintenance of Fluency', but we reject such terminology out of hand. The optimistic view of continual change and development inherent in personal construct theory is far more appealing than this behaviourist concept, which implies keeping things the same, as if there were a universal end-product to the process of stuttering therapy.

A theory of relapse

Throughout this book we have looked to the psychology of personal constructs to explain the process of change and how best to facilitate therapeutic movement. We can do likewise when we attempt to explain why some clients regress after seeming to improve. The explanations offered by PCT are not specific to stuttering relapse, but may explain why people find change difficult and resort to former ways of structuring their views of the world.

In personal construct theory a disorder is defined as 'any personal construction which is used repeatedly in spite of consistent invalidation' (**Kelly**, 1955, p831). Focusing on why an individual may use constructs repeatedly to anticipate the future, when they have already failed to achieve their purpose, provides a fruitful line of inquiry.

(a) Slot movement versus reconstruction

Most frequently relapse can be explained in terms of the superficial nature of the changes that have been made. Speech therapists often collude with their clients' unidimensional view of the problem: that change from stuttering to fluency only involves the learning of fluency skills. Therapy is directed to the speech and not the person; change is quick and therapy seems effective. However, because behaviour has been changed without accompanying reconstruction, fluency is likely to be meaningless to the person and relapse seems inevitable. What are the processes that might force retreat to stuttering?

(b) Constructs of transition

Engaging in the process of change involves *aggression:* the active elaboration of one's perceptual field. Although the change is desired, the consequences of change may bring about unexpected surprises. For example, Keith asked a person on the street the way, and did so fluently. Immediately afterwards he felt as if he had disappeared: he became just one of thousands of ordinary people on the street. The absence of reactions to *Keith stuttering* left him lost in a void of meaningless implications. Keith was aware of a lack of structure in the situation and was experiencing *anxiety*.

Adults who stutter have faced a lifetime of trying to predict when they will stutter in order to reduce anxiety. Our experience leads us to believe that people who stutter have a need for certainty and predictability. Because speaking is one of the most important ways of presenting ourselves, it is understandable that people who stutter become focused on speech and translate *all* their uncertainties into anxiety about stuttering. Their ways of construing themselves in relation to others may narrow down to such an extent that they peep at the world through a keyhole of anxiety. When faced with uncertainty, they may choose to concentrate really hard on speech in an effort not to stutter. Such an effort frequently results in stuttering, but the person may believe that not enough effort to be fluent was made and he therefore tries even harder next time.

Hence stuttering can be viewed as a disorder which provides a way of structuring reality, despite the fact that the effort not to stutter has been repeatedly invalidated. If the experience of anxiety is overwhelming we are forced to make a choice as to how to deal with it, and people who stutter keep choosing to put more and more effort into concealing their stuttering.

Therapy can be very *threatening* to some clients, especially when the implications of change involve them in core reconstruction. The subsystem of constructs to do with stuttering may be invalidated by therapy, leaving the person feeling anxious. When clients become aware of impending comprehensive change they may hang on to old structures for dear life. The speed with which fluency can be induced in a clinical setting may be very threatening for some clients.

When a person has stuttered since childhood, and stuttering becomes part of the core structure, to speak fluently may result in the experience of *guilt:* 'I am no longer myself if I don't stutter'. Through speaking fluently, core role structure has been lost, and again the lack of implications of fluency may leave the person feeling anxious.

Anxiety is the thread running through the dimensions of transition. On its own, anxiety usually implies that events cannot be construed by existing constructs. When anxiety is the result of threat or guilt, the experience may be even more overwhelming. Anxiety may lead to movement in any one of three directions.

1 **Hostility:** When people experience anxiety that is intolerable, and is a result of their own social experimentation, they may perseverate in order to validate their original anticipations (**Kelly**, 1955, p884). For example, Sheila decided it was time for her to get a job. She was in the middle of therapy and was making reasonable progress. She was sensing that one of the outcomes of therapy was that she would have to get a job, because she could no longer hide behind her stuttering. Without consultation, she hastily chose a job which involved demonstrating cookery, and which threw her into three of her most highly feared situations: groups, new people and having to say specific words. Of course she stuttered, and spent many sessions discussing her problems with her job. In the end she quit: her husband forced her to do so because she was not sleeping and was not her usual happy self. Her prediction that she could not go out to work because of stuttering had been validated.

2 Constriction: The movement towards constriction is another way of avoiding anxiety. People make their world manageable by restricting it to events which are construable and understandable. For example, Mary goes to college as a mature student and is confronted by a swirl of events that take her breath away. Being a student involves talking, arguing, acting on beliefs, socialising and so on, which are all new and anxiety-provoking situations for her. Rather than joining in, Mary pre-empts and says to herself: 'I am here to study, and nothing else'. From that moment on she studies with a vengeance. She is always in the library or at home working: she talks to virtually no one. She has made the situation manageable by constricting her world to studying and chooses to ignore student life for the time being.

3 Aggression: 'There are some persons who are distinguished by their greater tendency to set up choice points in their lives and then to make their elaborative choices' (**Kelly**, 1955, p509). Aggression is a solution to anxiety. If anxious people can take the courageous step of seeking out areas of confusion, testing potentially useful constructs and abandoning irrelevant ones, we may call them aggressive. For example, when Jonathan learned to listen to other people he found he could be much more spontaneous in his replies than previously, when he was busy thinking about what he was going to say next.

(c) Invalidation

Because many people who stutter live a cautious life, forever trying to control the amount of conflict or confusion they encounter, they may find that dealing with invalidation as a result of experimentation is very difficult. Already the years of stuttering have provided them with massive invalidation, and they may not feel able to handle yet more in therapy. Therapy poses the threat of invalidating core structures. Often we ask clients to be most aggressive on their weakest frontiers. We may be exposing them to invalidation of constructs that are in the process of being developed, or validating their negative view of themselves as being unable to change. Neither alternative is particularly satisfactory.

(d) Centrality of stuttering

As long as the *stuttering—fluency* construct remains one of the most highly elaborated ways of making sense of self in relation to others, it may govern the person's interpersonal behaviour and swings from one extreme to the other are likely. When this construct is loosened from its constellation, rendered impermeable and finally discarded, then the person may find other ways of construing role relationships. As indicated above, the more central or core this structure is, the more of a threat is posed by its abandonment: it is likely to be very resistant to change.

Summary

Clients may relapse for many reasons. The most obvious reason is that reversion to stuttering is the only pathway open to them when the implications of fluency evoke anxiety, threat or guilt. When newly formed structures are invalidated, the person may abandon these in favour of previously used constructions.

Continuing the process of change

This discussion will cover the sorts of problems people who stutter may have 'left over' once they have worked through the phases described in *chapters 6 and 7*. These problems may obstruct the continuing process of change. Some suggestions will be made as to how to deal with these. The contents of this section will also be useful for those clients who have returned to therapy after a break, perhaps because they are experiencing problems with speaking or wish to embark on further changes with the help of a therapist. The problems under discussion do not constitute a complete list of what might be on the agenda at this stage of therapy, but we hope that the methods and ideas discussed here, and in previous chapters, will enable therapists to deal with most of the problems that they encounter.

Problems that people bring to therapy

One way to approach this discussion is to consider the different problems that people may present in the later stages of therapy. We need to appraise the order of change that has occurred as well as the problems that continue to exist. It is probably safe to say that any lasting change that occurs as a result of weekly therapy originates from a change in attitudes or beliefs. It is usually not possible for someone to change a well-established pattern of behaviour by conscious control when therapy is limited to one session a week. However, if clients manage to change their attitudes as a result of careful exploration and experimentation, it is possible for behaviour to change spontaneously. During intensive therapy both first and second order change may occur; however, it is only through a detailed discussion that we can learn about the nature and extent of second order change. This means that when someone finds themselves stuck or at worst returning to the way they were, we should not make assumptions about the degree and type of change based upon length or frequency of previous therapy. All of the techniques that have already been described are useful when exploring these problems.

The problems or issues that are raised at this stage of therapy may be grouped as follows:

(i)   Problems centred around speech such as a decrease in fluency which may also be accompanied by an increase in avoidance and strong reactions to stuttering.
(ii) Problems centred around core constructs.
(iii) Problems involving role construing.
(iv) The threats posed by aggression.

The discussion below covers each of these areas separately and ways of tackling the problems are suggested. An increase in stuttering is likely to be a component of all the problems clients experience at this stage. Certainly, if our experience is valid, stuttering is always part of the complaint. By careful interviewing, we need to find out where the problems lie and how to set the process of change in motion again.

The contents of such an exploratory interview might be as follows:

■ When does the client stutter more; that is, to whom are they speaking, what is the content, why has the interaction occurred, who started it, what feelings accompanied the interaction, what was at stake, were there observers and so on.

■ Does one experience of stuttering lead to more?

- If the client had not stuttered what difference would that have made?
- What does the client try to do about stuttering?
- In the client's estimation, what triggered stuttering?
- What did the client think and do immediately after stuttering?

The answers to these questions will enable the therapist to make hypotheses about whether stuttering resulted from lack of practice of the techniques; from a fundamentally poor view of self; from an inability to construe the listener or situation; or from the client's need to slow down the process of change. These hypotheses can then be tested in therapy. The procedures are likely to be similar to those described throughout this book, but take into account the fact that the client is more experienced in the approach and in speaking fluently. As the discussion changes from the general to the more specific, so it may be possible to identify problems that fall into any of the following categories.

(a) Problems centred around speech

When clients mention that their speech is not as it should be, our first task is to determine at what level change should be effected. If first order change will suffice, in other words more practice, then there is no point in tackling more complicated procedures. However, if the client is trying really hard to use the techniques and is failing consistently, then to prescribe more of the same serves only to maintain the problem.

For some clients a review of speech techniques makes perfect sense. For example, clients who have made good use of first order change in the past and have gone on to change their attitudes are likely to use behaviour modification in similar ways a second time. Clients who have more of a cluttering problem than a stuttering problem may need to be reminded how to use the techniques to slow down and smooth out their speech. Their problem lies more in their disorganised speech than in inappropriate attitudes. A first order solution to the problem seems to be all that is needed.

Another example of situations where first order change seems useful is with clients who have had psychotherapy and have changed their attitudes to themselves and others. Despite their positive outlook on life they may retain some of the habits of stuttered speech and require straightforward speech work in order to become more fluent. An example of such a client is Luke, whose personal construct therapy was described in great detail by **Fransella** (1972). He found that he required some help with his speech and did well using prolonged speech. Changing his speech appeared to enable him to make better use of his change in attitudes.

Clients who have had some experience of block modification therapy often request more work on desensitisation. They may have expanded the situations in which they are willing to speak, but find that they are reluctant to stutter in these new situations, and may be avoiding or trying to conceal stuttering. Going through some of the same desensitisation procedures as mentioned in *chapter seven*, but taking account of the present circumstances, seems warranted. We have found setting up groups for advanced work on desensitisation to be very useful.

Desensitisation brings about second order change in most cases. We posit that, if clients use the ideas in desensitisation as techniques to increase fluency, they will fail, as they are taking a first order solution. The objective of desensitisation is to enable clients to stutter without feeling shame, guilt and anger. Such changes in attitude will only come about if clients can make personal sense of the experience of stuttering voluntarily, keeping eye contact, and so on.

Clients who have been taught prolonged speech and who then regress often ask to have the technique drummed into them again. They may have experienced a good stretch of fluency after such a course, and believe that if they can do it once, they can do it again. Experience has taught us that a second course of prolonged speech does not work. We would disagree with their view of what is needed and urge such clients to explore other options such as working on desensitisation. We would predict that they would be experiencing problems mentioned in the sections below, and that second order change is required.

(b) Problems centred around core construing

Core constructs subsume the essential self. Very often they involve constructs to do with *dependency*. In childhood, dependency is focused upon the parents, but as the child grows up dependencies are usually widely dispersed. Some people do not achieve this, and instead of meeting different needs in different relationships, they seek to have all their needs met in all relationships. It is as if they are seeking a parent figure: their hunger for love is insatiable.

When such a person seeks help as a client, therapists will be wise to proceed with extreme caution. 'Insight' into their undifferentiated dependencies may evoke a panic response and drive clients towards trying to become *independent*. A more appropriate way of helping clients is through active experimentation with more peripheral constructs. For example, one of our clients, called Raymond, showed signs of being very dependent on his therapist and certain friends. He was warm and grateful for every minute of therapy time, and became an ideal client. He worked really hard at reconstruing, but only in the context of therapy. There were always excuses about why experimenting outside therapy was impossible. It looked as if therapy would continue indefinitely. After various other alternatives to bring about change failed, the therapist presented Raymond with a problem for him to solve. She said that, in order to deal with some of the deeper problems which he wanted to explore, it was important that he had some context in which to relate to strangers. What could he suggest? In his efforts to please the therapist, Raymond chose to find himself a job. No sooner had he done so than he discovered that work met some of his needs so well that he no longer felt so dependent on the therapist. Because he had an area of stability and validation in his life we could now concentrate on dealing with his problem of dependency.

Readers may wonder why the experiment was set up in this particular way. The answer is quite simple. Raymond was refusing to experiment with his friends and family. To have accused him of not co-operating would have been very invalidating. Introducing the concept of strangers was a solution to this. On the surface, the experiment did not seem to be dealing with dependency issues, yet in fact it provided a context for Raymond to discover that dependency needs can be met in various ways. The solution to dealing with dependencies in therapy is to help the client to disperse rather than eliminate these needs.

Another problem which is related to core construing is that of *depression*. In personal construct theory terms, there are similarities in the ways of structuring life favoured by people who are depressed and by those who stutter. In both instances the symptom reduces the number of choices available and determines behaviour. **Rowe** (1983, p1) views depression as 'a prison where you are both the suffering prisoner and the cruel jailer'. In order to build the prison you must hold the following six opinions as if they were 'Real, Absolute and Immutable Truths'.

1 No matter how good and nice I appear to be, I am really bad, evil, valueless, unacceptable to myself and other people.

2 Other people are such that I must fear, hate and envy them.

3 Life is terrible and death is worse.

4 Only bad things happened to me in the past and only bad things will happen to me in the future.

5 It is wrong to get angry.

6 I must never forgive anyone, least of all myself. (p15)

If we consider each of these opinions in relation to stuttering, some of the similarities become clear.

1 Many people who stutter sense a dichotomy between their inner and outer selves. Often it is described in terms of speaking: 'Even when I speak fluently I know that inside I'm a stutterer'. Many people dread others finding out that they stutter: they do not want their inner, unacceptable self to be found out. People who feel this way do not allow positive experiences to change their essentially low opinion of themselves, no matter how fluent, successful or loved they are. Nothing every provides sufficient proof of their worth to allow a more positive construction of self. Such people may have suffered severe and frequent invalidation as children, with their attempts to please the adults around them either being ignored or met with demands for greater achievement.

2 People are often *feared* by those who stutter because they are seen to cause stuttering. Strangers, people in authority, people who ask direct questions, people who are unpredictable, and so on, are all to be feared. People who do not stutter are seen as leading problem-free lives and therefore are *envied*. If we choose to *hate*, we deny ourselves love and close friendship, which carry the risks of rejection or hurt. Stuttering can create a wall between people and hence reduce the chances of closeness and the risk of pain. If stuttering interfered with experimenting with relationships during the teens, then the risks for the adult are even greater. Not all people who stutter are socially isolated, but many do lead quite restricted lives, limiting themselves to only a few trusting relationships and viewing most other people with suspicion.

3 In Rowe's discussion of beliefs about life and death she stresses the difference between those who cope and those who do not. The difference is not between their actual belief systems, for example atheism, Christianity, Judaism or Hinduism, but whether their beliefs give them courage and optimism or whether they lead to fearfulness and pessimism:

> People who cope with their lives hold metaphysical beliefs which liberate or at least do not impede them. People who do not cope have beliefs which serve to trap them in a life of misery. (p38)

Stuttering may keep misery at bay since the person can live in hope that fluency will bring satisfaction to life. This makes fluency not only desirable but also dangerous, since it may force the person to try out their fantasy. If fluency does not bring about happiness, the person may have to reconstrue

176

their beliefs or constrict and face depression. The hostile choice would be to revert to stuttering, which prevents reconstruction. Understanding a person's metaphysical beliefs may explain relapse.

4 It is unfortunate that many of us remember our failures and unpleasant experiences more easily than the good ones. People who stutter have a very good memory for bad speaking experiences and the fluent times pass unnoticed. When they consider speaking experiences it is often only bad ones that can be recalled. On occasion we have introduced a ground rule in evening class groups whereby only good speaking experiences may be reported. At first this request is greeted with silence and then denial that there have been any good speaking experiences. Slowly positive experiences emerge, but often in very brief almost dismissive terms. The elaboration of fluent speaking formed a major part of **Fransella's** (1972) therapy, to good effect.

There is a time and place for discussing bad experiences, for if these are not shared they may become engraved on the memory. They are lived through over and over again in the mind and very rarely are they discussed. We have found these discussions useful at the start of a course of therapy but, as people start to change, we would like them to look to their futures, and not their hurtful past.

Stuttering is surrounded by silence: people who stutter do not talk about it and certainly not to somebody who is fluent, unless they have a professional interest. Before silence is broken, bad experiences of stuttering can easily dominate a person's thinking so that the past is bigger and more significant than either the present or the future. In this way the past clouds the future rather than providing a framework of anticipation.

5 Many people who stutter, like many fluent speakers, feel it is wrong to express anger. Because we want to be liked, and we need others' approval, it is difficult to be angry. People who stutter have an additional problem. As we have mentioned, stuttering may lead to feelings of unworthiness and to the anticipation of rejection. Therefore they must make every effort to compensate for the fact that they stutter. A strong need to be liked by others makes it difficult to get angry. It may also be difficult to say no. It may then easily happen that people take on too much, demand too high a standard of themselves and then become resentful. This resentment cannot be expressed verbally because it is just this type of talking that many people who stutter find particularly difficult. Learning to be assertive and finding that people do not dislike you can be liberating for someone who stutters. Expressing anger without loss of control helps to externalise frustrations and disappointments and so reduces the need for silent self-recrimination.

6 The silent recriminations that so many people who stutter engage in are a part of not being forgiving. Such people get caught in a situation where nobody wins: on the one hand, if they are *doing* the stuttering, that cannot be forgiven, and if the listeners have somehow *caused* the stuttering, they cannot be forgiven either. Every speaking situation can become a test of their value as a person and every stutter the proof of failure. These failures are then remembered.

Our attempt to fit stuttering into Rowe's model of depression leads us into the problems of stereotyping and there are dangers in this. The most serious problem is that only proof of the model's preciseness of fit will be entertained. We have included this discussion because it is our experience that progress with stuttering therapy can be halted when clients are depressed. When a client is basically pessimistic about self and life it is unlikely that long-term changes in speaking will occur. Success in therapy would challenge the client's view of self and hence bring about changes in core construing. It is unlikely that symptomatic therapy would prepare the client for the threat and anxiety that fluency would bring. Alternatively the depressed client may make progress but then regress when the next bout of depression occurs.

Support for the notion that depression may contribute to some clients' problems with change is provided in a study by **Price** (1987), who found a higher level of depression and trait anxiety among a group of 34 stuttering adults than would be expected in fluent speakers. She discovered a cluster of variables that may well have implications for progress in therapy. An external locus of control (**Rotter**, 1966) correlated with poor attitudes towards communication (**Andrews and Cutler**, 1974), greater levels of speech anxiety (**Brutten**, 1975) and higher levels of depression (**Beck** *et al*. 1961).

The locus of control refers to the person's beliefs about who controls their life: themselves (internal locus) or events and other people (external locus). It does not take much imagination to think of some of the implications that these beliefs have for therapy. When stuttering is coupled with depression we must decide which problem deserves priority and who is the most appropriate person to work with the client. Therapists with additional training may well feel able to tackle both the depression and the speaking problem. This is probably ideal since it helps the client to acknowledge the relationship between the two problems. When the depression and stuttering are viewed separately a vicious circle may interfere with progress—If I didn't stutter I wouldn't be depressed and if I wasn't depressed I wouldn't stutter. Also, if the two problems are being dealt with in very different ways by two different therapists, then they may end up working against each other and so separate therapy is only advisable when there is close contact between the two therapists.

It is not possible to review all the approaches to depression, but the approach outlined by **Rowe** (1983) may be helpful for clients whose depression is relatively mild. We would recommend referral of clients who are contemplating suicide. Rowe discusses ways of leaving the prison of depression and these largely follow on from the 'opinions' presented earlier. They are:

1 Don't play the 'Yes, but . . .' game.

2 Treat yourself kindly.

3 Put pills in your power.

4 Create a peaceful place within yourself.

5 Risk putting some trust in yourself and others.

6 Find someone to talk things over with.

7 Discover there's nothing wrong with seeing the funny side of things.

8 Dare to explore new ways of thinking and doing. (Chapter 7)

It is reassuring to note that, although half of the sample in the **Price** (1987) study were depressed, none of them were seriously so. If this is true for people who stutter in general, then it may be that the stuttering and depression may be maintained by similar ways of thinking.

(c) Problems with role construing

Some situations prove difficult, that is, they lead to stuttering, because the client cannot make useful predictions. The events lie outside the person's construct system, leading to anxiety. Probably these difficult situations have always precipitated anxiety and so it is by focusing on speech that the person regains some degree of predictive ability. By trying not to stutter, even though this may result in stuttering, the situation is brought back into the scope of the person's construct system, and so anxiety is reduced. The looks of embarrassment, the shortening of the conversation and so on, are predictable (**Fransella**, 1972). If clients were not so concerned about other people's reactions, they would probably not stutter so severely.

Because many clients use a constellation of constructs that cluster with *stuttering—fluency* they frequently believe that their listeners have the same ways of making sense of them. Clients are unable to contemplate other people's constructs until they have elaborated the meaning of these constructs for themselves. When they can place themselves as an element within the range of convenience of these new constructs, then they are likely to make better sense of people they speak with. The ways in which we construe ourselves influence the ways in which we construe others, and therefore work on self and role construing should go hand in hand. We tend to think that others think as we do, since this is the only way of thinking we have at our disposal. It may be very difficult to accept that others are not always as interested in us as we are in them.

This raises the interesting issue of validation. Our ways of making sense of other people need to be validated. Clients who speak fluently for the first time sometimes find that they cannot make sense of the seeming absence of reactions to themselves. By way of illustration consider a man who is terrified of a bat in his bedroom. His wife points out to him that the bat has no interest in him. The man says that he finds it difficult to believe that something he is so frightened of is essentially unaware of his existence. It may be very invalidating to acknowledge that the source of our fear is uninterested in us. The parallels with stuttering are evident: the person who stutters spends many long hours contemplating the people who are frightening, and may be very disappointed to learn that these people are not likewise engaged in dreaming up new ways of being intimidating.

It follows that therapy should aim to help clients make predictions that can be validated. However this is not enough to ensure lasting change: the validated predictions must be discussed and elaborated so that clients can incorporate these different ways of construing into their personal systems. Isolated successes will not help a person to replace well-used but limiting constructs with new, permeable ones. The activities listed below can all be used to discover different ways of making sense of hitherto difficult people or events.

Reconstruing a 'difficult' person [*]

First, the 'difficult' person is described in as much detail as possible by the client. Sometimes it becomes apparent that the main difficulty is that the client knows nothing about the person and cannot make any guesses. This may happen even when the problem person is encountered frequently, since the client is so anxious that the focus of attention is always on themselves. If this is the case, then it is worth spending time trying to formulate a picture of the person and setting suitable tasks to enable a fuller description at the next session.

---

[*] This procedure was introduced to the authors during a workshop run by Peggy Dalton.

179

The description should help clarify what it is about the person that bothers the client and also why that person is so significant in the client's life. Often the person is difficult because the client construes *easy and difficult* people on the basis of one or two discriminations. For example, Patrick had difficulty talking with people who were *older* than himself and also when the topic was *serious*. He had managed well when with fellow students, but was very anxious now that he had started work and was having to deal with people of all ages. Exploration of the implications of age and seriousness helped Patrick understand more about this particular difficulty.

The next step is to find some way for the client to construe and hence approach the difficult person that does not involve using constructs that previously led to stuttering. Preferably the way chosen should allow the client to use current skills. A client was dreading Christmas at her brother's house because of her sister-in-law's father. This man was a very successful surgeon, while the client was a nurse and so she felt inferior on account of her stutter and also because of the status of nurses in relation to consultant surgeons. She had never overcome her anxiety sufficiently to really notice much about the man as an individual, even though she got on well with her sister-in-law and wanted to be incorporated into the family. After much discussion it was decided that this Christmas the client would try to discover what the father had in common with his daughter. In order to help her get started in a positive way she was to concentrate on making the father feel welcome and comfortable, two things she was excellent at doing in a work context. In this way her ability to construe her sister-in-law was utilised, as were her skills as a nurse. This type of experiment is likely to lead to second order change: instead of focusing on better ways of controlling her stuttering, the problem has been reframed in such a way that a different approach is possible.

Whatever experiments are agreed upon it is essential that they are followed up in therapy. If clients find a better way of construing their 'difficult' person then this should help with some of the other people whom they find difficult. Exploration of the implications of the experiment should enable clients to incorporate these ways of construing into their construct systems. It will usually take about one hour to formulate an experiment involving a new way of relating to a problem person. Ideally, clients should choose to reconstrue people whom they see regularly, so that experimentation can follow the session.

Enactment

The value of enactment depends very much upon the way it is presented and used. Kelly differentiates between role play and enactment. In role play the aim is to be convincing in the role of another person. Acting the part of another does not have any value in this context since we know that people who stutter will be fluent under such circumstances and that this does not lead to fluency in real life. In contrast, enactment is based on role constructs: clients are asked to behave 'as if' they were another person. It is first and foremost an exercise in construing others, and the enactment is the outcome of that understanding. In enactment clients are asked to exchange parts before the enactment is discussed to experience the interchange from more than one perspective.

For example, if a client is to enact the role of a successful manager, what constructs are likely to be important to a manager at work? How will these discriminations influence behaviour? Probably we need to elaborate our construing of the manager a little more: is the client to be a paternalistic manager; or an assertive manager; or perhaps someone who gets things done by encouraging others to take responsibility? As these aspects of the role are explored, the client is being encouraged to elaborate his construing of managers, whom he may have previously construed mainly in terms of superiority and stuttering.

Many people who stutter have difficulty with 'authority figures'. Enactment encourages clients to begin to construe such people propositionally and to abandon pre-emptive constructs to do with status and social position. In the example above, the client was encouraged to think like a manager and to behave accordingly. He would also have had the opportunity to experience another person in the role of manager and this will have increased his understanding even further. Had this client been asked to role play a manager, he might have done so successfully on the basis of his previous construing and acted the part of a person who is full of their own importance and difficult to communicate with. Role play would not have led to reconstruing the *person* who is the manager.

It is usually obvious when enactment has a sense of significance to the participants, as opposed to being merely acted out. Sometimes, when people first attempt enactment, they cannot help but act. However, with experience and increased trust, most people are able to get into roles eventually. The responsibility is very much with the therapist to select appropriate scenes for enactment.

Some of the other helping professions use enactment to a greater extent than in speech therapy training. We found that use of such techniques as a student is of tremendous value and practical experience is perhaps an essential prerequisite to confident and appropriate use of enactment in therapy. Once the skills necessary for successful enactment have been developed the therapist has a technique that can be used for a variety of purposes. Some of these are given below and therapists are encouraged to add to the list as their experience grows.

- As practice prior to a real-life event.
- For desensitisation: the client's fears, as well as more common responses, can be explored.
- To experiment with different approaches towards people and situations.
- To experience the position of the person in the other role.
- To share the different constructions of the situation that each person places upon it. The people involved in the enactment and those observing can all contribute.
- To share evaluations of behaviour during the enactment.

Another bonus derived from enactment is that the ensuing discussion tends to be meaningful: people have shared an experience and they are often eager to present their opinions and thoughts about it. Clients may find their views of things challenged, but protected by the safety of the therapy room and in the context of viable alternatives. The experience tends to linger in the mind of the protagonist and this can be a real help when the actual situation arises.

If a video-recorder is available it can be used to help with the discussion stage. If people are very nervous about enactment they may not be able to construe much of what occurs. Watching the event immediately afterwards allows the players to relive the part but in a more reflective frame of mind. Although groups of about four people are ideal, enactment can still be used effectively in individual therapy and in larger groups.

Before concluding our discussion on enactment, we would like to emphasise that it is a very powerful tool. The only way that therapists can acquire experience is by experimenting themselves. Where therapists are working as part of a team they may find it helpful to enact the role of some of their cleints with a colleague taking the part of the therapist. Not only will this further therapists' understanding of their clients, but it will serve to desensitise therapists to being watched. When first using enactment with clients, the following points may be useful:

- present the idea of enactment as an invitation to explore a situation, rather than as something clients have to be good at;
- keep the enactments brief;
- ask people to stay in role no matter whether other people do or not;
- at the end of the enactment, especially if the protagonists have been asked to enact 'undesirable' parts, it is useful to ask people to free themselves of the role by saying who they are. For example, 'I am Celia, speech therapist'.

Extending role construing through experimentation

We are often surprised by the way in which intelligent, perceptive people can convince themselves that stuttering is the only insoluble human problem. Perhaps on another level it is not so surprising: probably we have all been taught that if we work hard and try hard, we will get what we want in life. A popular view of poverty, mental illness and unemployment is that those who suffer such misfortunes do, in some way, deserve it. Most people who stutter put enormous effort into speaking fluently, often to no avail. In addition, they often lead 'good lives': it is easy to be blatantly unkind to people if you are fluent; it is also easier to reach a powerful position. Some clients feel as if they are undeserving victims of stuttering and their progress may be hindered by resentment. They feel themselves trapped by a stutter that behaves rather like an evil demon: no matter how good they are, it is always there either punishing or threatening to punish them. To make matters worse, it insists on meting out punishment in front of others and so both pain and humiliation are experienced.

During the early stages of therapy the client may have neither the inclination nor the fluency to talk to other people about their problems. However, as therapy progresses this can be an extremely useful exercise and much can be gained by setting clients the task of asking others about personal problems and how they deal with them. First, clients are encouraged to contemplate the fact that others do have problems; second, they need to think quite carefully about other people before deciding whom to approach; third, in deciding how to make the approach they will need to take account of the other person's feelings; fourth, in order to do the task the client has to engage with another person. If all goes well the client may learn about the following:

- At least one example of a problem not concerned with speaking;
- How the person goes about dealing with the problem;
- How successful they are; *and*
- How they feel about it.

Quite often a conversation like this will lead to a discussion about the client's stuttering, therefore providing an opportunity to talk openly about it without feeling inferior by virtue of having a problem. When the task of finding out about other people's problems and their ways of dealing with them is set as a group exercise, useful discussions may follow. An exercise in understanding others begins to prepare the person who stutters for the reality of new problems replacing old ones. The client may see that a positive approach or philosophy of life is more useful than an armoury of tricks designed to deal with only one sort of problem. When clients engage in conversations about problems with people who have found ways of dealing with them, they are encouraged to take a broader perspective than usual.

Frameworks for understanding other people

We find that personal construct theory offers us a framework within which to make sense of ourselves and the people we encounter. Within this framework, behaviour is seen as an experiment based on personal constructs. To understand another person we are required to construe their construction processes. While this concept is central to our beliefs, we are about to set it aside and describe an alternative framework that may be helpful in interpersonal transactions. There are a variety of approaches towards encouraging *assertive behaviour* and we shall consider just one. We shall not be talking about 'assertiveness training' since this would conflict too seriously with our approach.

In our stuttering therapy the aim of working on increasing assertiveness is to find ways of relating to people other than through the dominating *stuttering—fluency* construct. The client is encouraged to stereotype transactions, but this is viewed as a short-term expedient. The construct *assertive—unassertive* is an interesting one, since it is seldom used by people who stutter and has different implications from more common ways of construing behaviour as aggressive, superior, strong and so on. Therefore it provides the client with an alternative way of construing behaviour that has no difficult implications and does not encourage 'slot-rattling' (moving from one end to the other of a construct dimension and back again). Finally, we can justify using an assertive model with those clients who have difficulty in standing up for themselves, because it offers ways of behaving that are neither over-aggressive nor compliant.

Cox and Dainow (1985, p82) describe the assertive person as someone who is able and willing to evaluate, negotiate and communicate. The message that underlies the content of assertive communication is: 'This is what I think; this is what I feel; this is how I evaluate the situation. I'm interested in what you think, and will respect your right to your own opinions. I'm willing to negotiate with you'. An assertive response contains these elements presented in such a way that communication is facilitated. The authors stress that the aim is not always to be assertive, but to have some choices about the way we behave in relation to others.

Typically assertive responses are contrasted with *aggressive, indirectly aggressive* and *passive* responses. An example of each of these responses to a particular problem is given below:

> You feel unhappy that you're always the one to empty the rubbish bins for the house, and you want to divide general household tasks more evenly.
> 1. You get angry and accuse your partner of being a slovenly pig.
> 2. You complain about the pressures of work, how tired you are, and how near you are to a nervous breakdown.
> 3. You feel guilty for even thinking about discussing what you think of as clearly *your* job.
> 4. You set time aside to discuss the division of labour and state clearly what you'd like. (p80)

(1 = aggressive; 2 = indirectly aggressive; 3 = passive; 4 = assertive)
We suggest that therapists explore this model with their clients. The

four categories seem to help people to reflect upon their own styles of behaviour. Setting up enactments using each of the different modes of behaving enables clients to test predictions and make decisions as to how to vary their own behaviour in the future. One advantage of this model is that the responsibility for the style of communication is given to the speaker. People who stutter often feel that stuttering affects the way people behave towards them. Being more assertive might not always guarantee fluency, but it should engender a sense of choice which stuttering often undermines. This model of assertiveness aims to help people clarify the messages they give so that resentment and misunderstanding are reduced. The emphasis upon *effective communication* rather than *control* fits very well with the general orientation of our therapy.

Some people spontaneously become more assertive as they become more fluent, but many others make mistakes and feel disheartened. For example, Desmond made extensive use of a role construct which correlated with stuttering and fluent speaking, and presented him with a double bind. The construct was *arrogant—humble*. When stuttering, he felt humble, but when fluent, he would become increasingly arrogant. This would elicit very negative reactions from his friends, and he would feel squeezed back along both constructs to shameful stuttering. The alternative to being arrogant or humble lay in finding a way for Desmond to be more sensitive to other people's feelings, which neither pole of his original construct offered. Being assertive provided such a possibility, and behavioural experiments to test this construct were set up.

The ability to be assertive comes from developing a set of hypotheses to be tested in the social sphere. Learning to *behave* assertively does not imply that such construing has taken place. 'Whistling in the dark' does not mean that the person is unafraid. Therefore the task at hand is to help clients to elaborate the meaning of being assertive, to construe the difference it may make to their lives and to abandon former ways of interacting. The assertive person makes the most of themselves (**Cox and Dainow**, 1985).

(d) The threat of aggression

Change can be exhilarating. To have a sense of choice, to feel that anything is possible, to be aware that self can be reinvented is powerfully intoxicating. The object of therapy is change: usually, we complain that there is too little change, but sometimes there can be too much!

When clients who stutter start to move in therapy they may develop a sense of urgency to make up for lost time that leaves the therapist breathless. Suddenly, jobs are changed, new relationships started: things seem to be happening too fast. Action seems to precede thinking and collapse seems inevitable.

What might be happening psychologically? First, the person might be construing self on all the positive poles within their system for the first time. These might be relatively unelaborated, and so full circumspection is not possible before decisions are made. Clients pre-empt and choose impulsively and, because of the importance of the issues involved, may have to reconstrue themselves very rapidly. Take the example of Sheila, who launched herself into the threatening situation of finding a job that involved demonstrating cookery. She found that her relationship with her husband was threatened because it was founded on her dependence on him. If she were to become financially independent would that lead to emotional independence, and would she then be able to maintain the relationship? In this case, both parties felt threatened. Sheila resorted to hostility: she said that she could not hold down a job because of her speech. Her husband opted for the right to protect her and asked her to quit because she was not her usual happy self.

The therapeutic strategy which is deemed to be most helpful in these circumstances is controlled elaboration. This is similar to the elaboration of fluency described in *chapter seven*. Clients are asked to expand their view of themselves now that they have changed and to experiment to ensure that the new ways of construing self are useful for anticipating events. Another strategy for elaborating the person's construing is to ask clients to write a self characterisation or to complete a grid. Comparing the elements *as I am now* with *as I used to be* not only measures the extent of change, but helps the client to construe the present more realistically. This type of activity focuses their attention on the way they construe and serves to slow down active experimentation.

Many of the other examples we have quoted illustrate that one person's aggression may be another person's threat. This is particularly so in the context of relationships or families, and calls upon therapists to develop skills in couple counselling or family therapy. Sometimes, as therapists, we are faced with difficult decisions: we become aware that a person will lose their relationship if they continue to change. Where does our loyalty lie? Must we choose to help the client, regardless of who else falls by the wayside? Can we help the other parties through the client? Do we insist that all people involved come for therapy together? Each of these choices is valid in particular circumstances, and needs to be negotiated with the client who first seeks therapy. We have found it useful to extend the invitation to family members, even in the context of direct work on speech. The offer is seldom accepted, but the fact that it is discussed at home, and that families know they are welcome, may be helpful in itself.

Although people change by being aggressive and by actively elaborating their construct systems, change in therapy needs to be orchestrated. Therapists need to take account of the risks of change for their clients, and to attempt to set up experiments that can be validated. This involves being constantly aware of the context in which the person is seeking to change.

Terminating therapy

Ways of terminating therapy in the group context have been discussed in *chapter eight*. Similar issues are involved when ending therapy with an individual client. Because we are not able to cure stuttering in adults, how do we know when to stop therapy? Who terminates therapy: the therapist or the client? This leads to a further problem: if we do know it is time to stop therapy, how do we go about doing it?

Clients may terminate therapy for many reasons. They may feel that they have achieved their goals and can manage on their own. They may leave because therapy has become very threatening for them. Perhaps circumstances have changed, removing some of the troublesome elements from their lives, so that they no longer have to face the difficulties they used to have. Sometimes time and money constraints determine the end of therapy. Some clients find therapy humiliating: they feel they ought to be able to solve their own problems. Occasionally clients feel that they have learned the methodology of change and are able to be self-directing.

The reasons that therapists may have for terminating therapy are usually that the goals have been achieved and that the client is able to function autonomously. Sometimes time limits are set at the start of therapy and, as the end approaches, termination procedures can be initiated. Setting time limits is very difficult, because it is not always possible to specify the time needed to effect certain changes. Neither party may feel that termination is appropriate, and this may be experienced as a failure by either or both participants.

If the therapist decides to end the relationship, she will need to check that she is doing so for the good of the client and not herself. Many therapists resent clients who become dependent or fail to progress. As we have indicated in earlier chapters, the therapist has responsibility for these issues. Obviously, if therapy is getting nowhere, there is little point continuing with it, and the therapist may wish to refer the client elsewhere or terminate all intervention.

Brammer and Shostrom (1968) suggest the following steps and methods of closure:

1 *Verbal preparation:* This involves talking about the fact that therapy is drawing to a close because the client has achieved the goals specified at the start of therapy.

2 *Summary statement:* The client and therapist review together the course of therapy and may each write and share their view of what has happened. Such reports should also be anticipatory: they should include predictions about the future, maybe at a very specific level. For example, 'The first thing I will do is arrange to join a public speaking class'. More general statements, such as, 'I feel more able to talk to new people now' are also appropriate.

3 *Follow-up sessions:* It is helpful to leave the door open for future sessions. Clients may wish to return to tell the therapist that all is well, or to discuss new problems that were not anticipated. The alternative to this is to refer the client to another therapist, if there are outstanding problems that cannot be dealt with in the context of the current relationship.

4 *Formal leave taking:* The way in which the therapist says the final goodbye is very important. The client should leave feeling that the therapist has confidence in the client's ability to deal with the future. Therapists should be aware that it is often difficult to let a client go, and that their wishes to be part of the client's future should be dealt with in their own supervision.

Optimal functioning

What is the end-product of successful personal construct therapy? We start with Kelly's optimistic assertion that 'no one needs to be the victim of his biography' (p15). It is not our potential, but rather what we dare to do, that determines what we become. Change in therapy begins with the client attempting to answer the question, 'What are my immediate objectives?' The answer should precipitate the person into actions which challenge previously held definitions of self. The person sets out to be something that they are not. One of the immediate goals of therapy is to help clients evolve a construct system through which they can move towards their objectives. The ingredients of change are commitment and investment in the venture of life.

Who determines the end-product of therapy? Certainly not the therapist. Therapy provides people with an experience in which 'one person makes constructive use of another who has offered himself for that purpose. The professional skills of the therapist, as well as much of his repertory as an experienced human being, are brought into the transaction. He offers as much of both as he thinks can be used. But it is the client who weaves them into the fabric of his own experience' (**Kelly**, 1980, p21).

A person who functions optimally is one who 'is able to construe the world in such a way that predictions are, for the most part, validated. When invalidation *does* occur, the person deals with it by reconstruing' (**Fransella**, 1984, p133). Such a person faces the future with the sure knowledge that change is part of life.

PERSONAL GROWTH AND DEVELOPMENT OF THE THERAPIST

CHAPTER 10
PERSONAL GROWTH AND DEVELOPMENT OF THE THERAPIST

Are good therapists born or made?

Throughout this book we have elaborated Kelly's view of the person as self-creating: utilising cycles of experience to evolve personal theories about the world in which we live. 'Experience is made up of the successive construing of events. It is not constituted merely by the succession of events themselves' (**Kelly**, 1955, p73). As we observe the colourful pageant of life marching by, we note recurring themes and organise and reorganise our thinking to predict and thereby gain control over events. For example, during the course of training, speech therapists are supplied with many constructions of the problem of stuttering. It is only in clinical practice that these can be tested, but unless therapists are prepared to reflect on their experience they may not evolve a subsystem of personal constructs that enable them to develop better strategies for helping people who stutter. Therapy may continue to be governed by 'borrowed' constructs: knowledge may not become personal.

In order to learn and to grow, we need to construe our experience. This involves putting our hypotheses on the line, conducting experiments and reviewing the findings. We may have to discard invalidated constructs and replace them with ideas that have greater predictive accuracy. In order to make good use of our personal constructs we may need to examine the hierarchical structure and organisation of our systems and try to minimise inconsistencies between constructs. For example, if our experience in life has taught us that people change by talking things through, we may find that adopting a rigid behavioural approach to stuttering would make us feel uneasy as a person. To quell the disquiet, we could either make people who stutter a special case, and do therapy that seems incompatible with our personal philosophy of life, or we could discard one of the conflicting ideas, whichever is least resistant to change. An example such as this demonstrates how we may incorporate ideas from our training into our personal systems and how important it can be to have self-understanding.

We are fully committed to the notion that therapists are self-created. Further, we believe that one of the responsibilities we have as therapists is to develop a system of constructs about therapy and about our roles as therapists. We need to develop constructs to do with understanding ourselves and our clients, and find ways of reflecting on that understanding. At the very least this involves being able to have an internal dialogue within oneself about therapy. The conversation-within-self may require therapists to formulate hypotheses about clients and, once these have been tested during sessions, to evaluate and revise their developing system of predictions about clients. At the very best, therapists will arrange to have supervision of their therapy with a colleague. Supervision, which is discussed in more detail below, helps therapists to develop ways of viewing their own therapy and therefore to change it. Having access to another therapist's personal construct system is likely to be a beneficial learning experience for therapists.

The exercises which follow are intended to enable therapists to conduct a conversation within themselves. This will involve making assumptions about therapy and stuttering explicit, and follows the process we have undergone ourselves in writing this book.

Exploration of assumptions underlying therapy

(a) Comparing and contrasting therapy with other activities

Consider the following elements:

- Reading a novel
- Talking to a close friend
- Discussing politics in a group of friends
- Helping an old person cross the road
- Planning games for a children's party
- Fixing a broken machine

Now find one way in which each of these elements is *similar* to doing therapy. Write down the contrast poles of each to define the construct. For example, Sarah finds *reading a novel* and *doing therapy* are similar in that they both involve *absorbing what someone else has to say*. The opposite of this might be *being self-absorbed*.

Next, find one way in which each of these elements is *different* from doing therapy. Again note the contrast poles. For example, Sarah finds *reading a novel* and *doing therapy* are different from each other in that reading *involves taking no responsibility for what happens* whereas therapy implies *taking responsibility for what happens*.

The twelve constructs thus elicited concern therapy and provide some understanding of how therapy is compared and contrasted with other activities. The similarities indicate some of the experience and/or attitudes from ordinary living that we bring to our work as therapists. The differences indicate the ways in which therapy seems different from ordinary life.

Looking at the list, mark the pole for each construct that you as a person prefer. Go through the list again, marking the preferred poles from the point of view of yourself as therapist. Now see if there are any incompatibilities. In the example above, suppose that as a person Sarah prefers *being self-absorbed*, but as a therapist she prefers *absorbing what someone else has said*. Awareness of this may help her growth as a therapist in that she would gain insight into why she finds therapy hard work. In the long term she may reconstrue and find that listening more attentively is beneficial to herself as a person, but in the meanwhile she is aware of what she has to 'switch on' when she enters work.

(b) Construing the process of change

Our task as therapists is to help people change. We may find changing ourselves very easy or very difficult. The exercises which follow should help therapists increase their awareness of the issues involved in change.

(i) Change over time

Draw a line on a piece of paper and mark off the years of your life from birth to the present. Using arrows to point to the time line, mark at least five events that have resulted in personal change. Very often the events that lead to change involve choice points in our lives: choosing a partner in life, choosing a career, choosing a political party, choosing to leave home, choosing a new hairstyle and so on.

Mark off at least five points on your time line where you chose not to change: for example, staying in the same job, giving a relationship a little more time, not moving house and so on.

Looking back at the points in your life when you felt that change was possible:

1 How did you make the decision leading to change?
2 What did you predict might happen?
3 How long did it take to make the decision?
4 What were the risks involved in making the choice?
5 What help did you have from others at the time?
6 How did you feel during the decision-making period?

What about the times when you felt you could not go through with changing?

1 What were the possibilities open to you?
2 What did you predict might happen?
3 What were the risks for you?
4 How did you make the decision not to change?
5 What were your feelings at the time?
6 What factors within yourself or your circumstances made change seem impossible?

The examples given above probably involved major life changes. Consider some of the smaller, less obvious ways in which you have tried to change, and reflect on how these changes came about, what it felt like during the process of change, and what losses and gains accrued to you as a result. Were other people involved? Did they notice anything different? Did they support you or feel you were wasting your time?

(ii) A small experiment with change

It is likely that the series of questions above has highlighted some of the issues involved in past changes that you have made in your life. But what is it like to plan change, monitor it and evaluate the results? We would like you to plan to change in some small, but nevertheless important way. We would like you to stick to your resolution to change for four to six weeks and to record your progress each week.

1 Choose some behaviour that you wish to change: for example, your eating habits, punctuality, reading a newspaper.
2 Identify what you see as 'the problem', that is, what you think you are doing wrong.
3 Identify the reasons you wish to change: what difference will it make?
4 Construct a plan of action:
   (a) what do you plan to do each day?
   (b) how are you going to monitor change?

(c) whom are you going to tell and/or involve?

(d) what leeway are you going to give yourself: what are your minimum and maximum targets each day?

5 How easy or difficult do you predict changing will be?

6 If you change in this way, what else about you will change?

7 Is there anyone who wants you to change?

8 Is there anyone who does not want you to change?

9 How will you know if you are doing a good job or a bad job?

10 What past experience of changing can you draw on to help you this time?

At the end of the four- to six-week period, review what has been learned about change and reflect on the predictions you made before you began.

(c) Assumptions about stuttering

The following exercises aim to access your implicit theories and feelings about stuttering. We call upon you to be completely honest with yourself: no one is watching! A good way to deal with 'problem' attitudes is to know what they are, so that you can change them.

(i) Attitudes to stuttering

All you know about a person is that they stutter. What else might they be like? Make a note of your answer to the question, and then take each attribute one at a time, and try to answer the following questions:

1 How do you know that . . . is typical of people who stutter?

2 Can you think of any person who stutters where this is not the case? How do you account for this?

3 Can you think of a person who does not stutter who has this trait? How do you account for this?

By the time you have completed this exercise, you will have challenged your way of construing people who stutter. Most speech therapists are willing to stereotype people who stutter, saying they are typically 'nervous, self-conscious, tense, sensitive, anxious, fearful, afraid, hesitant, insecure and intelligent' (**Turnbaugh, Guitar and Hoffman**, 1979, 22, pp37–45). But are we correct in doing so? Are we not merely borrowing constructs from the literature and from our teachers and colleagues?

We have made much of Kelly's view of the therapeutic relationship as being a joint venture, a partnership. Is it possible to accord equality and respect to clients whom we view so negatively? It is probable that speech therapists and people who stutter hold a more negative stereotype of stuttering than the rest of the population. The next exercise aims to explore this.

(ii) Stuttering and society

We would like to suggest that therapists explore the attitudes of the general public to stuttering, not in their capacity as therapists, but rather as members of the public themselves. The following tasks may be of use:

1 Telephone a job centre or employment agency and say you have a friend who stutters severely and ask about their chances of employment. Try a few places and ask about jobs which involve different amounts of talking.

2 Telephone a doctor, hairdresser and dentist and try and make an enquiry while stuttering yourself. Vary the severity of stuttering with each call.

3 If you happen to meet people who do not know you are a therapist, tell them about a person who stutters and try and draw out their opinions on stuttering.

4 Try stuttering while buying train tickets, shopping or asking someone the time.

We do not expect you to have an easy time of these tasks, but you will probably gain useful information about attitudes to stuttering that may confirm or challenge your own views.

5 In your capacity as a therapist, talk about stuttering to your friends and family. Ask them questions about its cause, its treatment, how they believe it affects people and why they think they do not stutter.

(iii) Theories about stuttering

What is your theory about stuttering? As an exercise write about your personal theory of stuttering covering the following areas:

1 Cause(s);

2 Development;

3 Variability: why stuttering varies from person to person and within each person on different occasions;

4 Maintaining factors: what keeps stuttering going once it is established?

5 Spontaneous recovery: why do 75 per cent of those who start stuttering stop by the age of 13?

Now classify your theory: is it psychological, physiological, neurological, a learned behaviour, or what? How does your theory influence your therapy?

(d) The therapeutic relationship

(i) Construing the relationship

Write down a list of six clients. If you only work with people who stutter, choose six, trying to pick some clients you get on well with and some you get on less well with. If you work with people with different speech problems, choose from your full case load. Now focus on your relationships with any two of these clients. *In what important way are these relationships (not clients) similar or different?*

Make a note of this pole and the contrast pole as well. Continue to elicit relationship constructs from different pairs of clients until the same themes keep cropping up. Add other clients if you wish to explore this area more broadly. The pool of constructs you have collected will be based on the ways you make sense of your therapeutic relationships.

Now mark the poles of each construct which describe your current relationships with clients most accurately. Check through the list once more and mark your preferred way of relating to clients. If there are discrepancies, what can you do to change things? You may like to compare notes with colleagues and decide what is ideal, what is practical and what is undesirable in a therapy relationship.

(ii) The relationship with families and children

The following list of questions by **Cunningham and Davis** (1985, p20) is useful for checking how your relationship with children and families is progressing. Answering most of the questions positively indicates that you are working in partnership with the family. If most of your answers are negative, you may need to consider why this is so.

194

1 Have I met the family?

2 Do I consider the child in the context of their family?

3 Do I have regular, two-way communication with the family?

4 Do I respect and value the child as a person?

5 Do I respect and value the family?

6 Do I feel the family has strengths to help the child?

7 Have I identified the parent's abilities and resources?

8 Do I always act as honestly as possible?

9 Do I give them choices about what to do?

10 Do I listen to them?

11 Have I identified their aims?

12 Do I negotiate with them?

13 Do I adjust according to the joint conclusions?

14 Do I assume they have some responsibility for what I do for their child?

15 Do I assume I have to earn their respect?

16 Do I make the assumption that we might disagree about what is important?

17 Do I believe they can change?

18 Have I tried to identify the parent's perceptions of their child?

(e) Why are you a therapist?

Have you considered why you have chosen to be a therapist? Are you in the therapy business because you are altruistic? Or have you made the choice because you 'want to work with people?' Even if the answers to these questions are affirmative, there are likely to be other motivations for choosing to be a helper.

Completing the following sentences may help you discover your personal motives for becoming a therapist:

As a speech therapist –

(a) I am becoming the kind of person who . . .
(b) My strengths are . . .
(c) My weaknesses are . . .
(d) What I need most from people is . . .
(e) What I give to people most of the time is . . .

(**Munro, Manthei and Small,** 1983, p21)

It may be helpful to ask a colleague to do the same exercise so that you can compare notes. You may like to consider how easy or difficult it was to complete the statements honestly. If you have probed deeply, you may find that therapy is fulfilling your needs as a person in particular ways. You may need to ask yourself where you can meet these needs other than in the therapy context, and to work towards finding alternative sources to this end.

(f) Further self-exploration

Before using some of the techniques described in *chapter two*, therapists may find it useful to try these out on themselves.

(i) Writing a self characterisation

The instructions for writing a character sketch appear on page 23. Write one or two of your own: as a person; as a therapist. Analyse what you have written following the instructions in *chapter two*, and assess the value of the exercise for yourself.

Having written many character sketches ourselves over the years, we have realised just how personal a document it can be. We suggest that therapists only request clients to write characterisations when their contents will be used in therapy. If therapy aims to teach a fluency technique and nothing else, a speech assessment at the start of therapy is probably all that is needed. If therapy is going to focus on the psychological aspects of stuttering, then a self characterisation is certainly warranted.

(ii) Eliciting, laddering and pyramiding of constructs

Some of the exercises above ask therapists to elicit constructs from themselves. These focus in the main on therapy. Therapists may find it useful to elicit constructs from elements drawn from other aspects of their lives. Again the procedures are described in *chapter two* on page 17.

It is very difficult to 'ladder' oneself. Experience in this important technique may be gained by involving a colleague or friend. Eliciting, laddering and pyramiding constructs from each other can be a rewarding experience and promote mutual understanding. It also provides an opportunity for feedback on technique. A word of caution: when working with a friend, it is very tempting to supply answers or to disagree with what your friend says. The same rules of credulous listening applies even though the context may be very different from the therapy exchange.

(iii) ABC model

Again the technique for exploring implicative dilemmas is described in *chapter two*. We suggest that you choose a construct where you are not on your preferred pole, and ask yourself about the advantages and disadvantages of each end of the construct. It might be useful to select a construct along which you would like to change: for example, losing weight, starting to study, or increasing self-awareness. If you have chosen to work through laddering and pyramiding with a colleague or friend, then you might try this procedure with them as well.

Although we are ending the section of self-exploration here, we hope that therapists will invent their own activities if need be to gain greater awareness of their values and assumptions which underly their work as therapists. The next section examines some of the skills which we believe foster good therapeutic practice.

The development of therapeutic skills

(a) Listening skills

Learning to listen is a complicated process involving much more than simply *hearing* what a person has to say. It involves awareness of self as well as the awareness of the spoken and unspoken cues from the speaker. The aim of listening in the therapeutic context is to enter the world of the client: to see things from their perspective. Different listening skills may be required at different times during the therapy process.

(i) The credulous approach

Kelly advises therapists to use the credulous approach to listening, especially in the first few sessions. We have found this approach useful whenever we feel we are not quite understanding what a client is telling us. The dictionary defines being credulous as 'tending to believe something on little evidence'

(*New Collins Concise Dictionary*, 1982), which is certainly implied by Kelly. He continues by urging us never to discard information given by the client because it does not quite fit our picture of what is wrong. Both the spoken and unspoken behaviour of the client conveys an intrinsic truth for the client. Clients will present us with their personal construction of events, which may or may not accord with the ways in which other people construe these same events. Our task as listeners is to absorb all the information, until such time as we have enough detail to formulate an overview of the problem or problems of our clients.

(ii) Attending skills

Attending skills involve listening with every fibre of your being. Body posture, movement and eye contact are all important markers of an attentive listener. A person wants to feel the other's psychological presence. Listening cannot be faked.

As an exercise, ask two colleagues to join you in exploring your attending behaviours. One person assumes the role of client, one the role of therapist and one acts as observer. The 'client' presents a problem, and the 'therapist' tries out two ways of behaving: first, listening as carefully as possible, and second, indicating lack of interest. Once everyone has taken on all three parts, discuss the feelings that accompany each style of listening from each of the three perspectives.

(iii) Following skills

Not only do we need to show that we are attending, we need to reduce our input to a minimum until we are clear as to how our clients are seeing things. We frequently use questions as a way of inviting a person to talk on some subject or other. We need to guard against questions being implicitly judgemental. For example, 'Did you stutter much this week?' Contrast this with a statement such as 'You look a bit harassed today. Would you care to talk about it?'

During a conversation the speaker is likely to respond well to minimal encouragers, which can be verbally or non-verbally given. Head-nodding, the ubiquitous 'uhuh' or a gentle probe such as 'then?' are all signs that the listener is following and interested. Silences are also useful ways of encouraging a person to talk. Many people, including therapists, have a low tolerance of silence. Working on this skill as a therapist can be extremely beneficial to a client who is having difficulty talking, provided it is not used aggressively. Practising these skills in ordinary conversation so that they are delivered naturally and do not sound stilted or obviously therapeutic may be helpful to therapists.

(iv) Reflecting skills

Reflecting skills afford therapists the opportunity of checking their understanding of what has been said by the client. This can be done by paraphrasing what the client has said, for example: 'Let me see if I have got that right. When you went to work the other day, you were feeling that you couldn't face your boss?'

In the same way, the therapist may summarise the chief points made during a long stretch of talking by the client. Summaries may also be used at the ends of sessions to highlight what was discussed. At times it is useful to ask the client to do this as it helps pull loose threads together so that the client can leave the session with some structure for coping with life outside.

Some approaches to therapy focus on feelings, and reflection is certainly a useful way to show clients that you understand and accept what they are saying. Again doing this in a natural way, without sounding robotic, requires practice. Styles differ between therapy approaches. Within some counselling approaches, therapists are taught to pick up feeling words, for example:

Client: I am furious with my brother for saying that.
Therapist: You feel furious.

We feel that this manner of responding is very stilted and prefer to acknowledge feelings or to anticipate them, for example:

Client: I just stood there, couldn't say a thing.
Therapist: It must have been pretty scary.

If reflections are offered tentatively, as one possible version of the situation, then they are likely to help the client to elaborate and understand their problem. If they are presented as the truth, they may block the therapeutic process.

(b) Developing interviewing skills

In the early stages of information gathering, the therapist is likely to ask many questions. How these are phrased is likely to influence the therapeutic relationship and probably the course of therapy.

As an exercise, record an initial interview session and note all the questions you asked. See which ones led you to greater understanding of the client's problem. Which questions were unnecessary? Which questions require rephrasing to be more effective? It is relatively easy for an interview to degenerate into an interrogation with too many questions being asked, where the questions are closed or leading and where there are too many 'why' questions. Certainly such questions help the therapist accumulate a great many facts, but do they help to understand the problem from the client's point of view?

Instead of expanding on the mistakes we all make, we would like to make some positive suggestions for obtaining sufficient information from a client to direct both client and therapist towards a solution. These techniques are useful, not only at the start of therapy, but also during the therapy process when a client wants to explore a particular problem in more depth.

(i) Controlled elaboration

For Kelly, controlled elaboration involves helping the client to convey the nature of the complaint to the therapist without getting lost in detail. Although it is offered as a way of getting information, Kelly recognises its therapeutic value. As a person elaborates their system, so the system is clarified. Relationships between constructs are made more explicit, and greater self-understanding is likely to be achieved.

Language is the chief tool of controlled elaboration and helps both client and therapist to pin things down. The therapist helps the client seek out the major ways of construing particular events, asking questions such as, 'What was important to you about that event?' For example, in discussing a talkative sister with a client, the following dialogue took place:

Client: My sister always used to get her own way.
Therapist: Whereas you . . .?
Client: I never did.
Therapist: Which would you have preferred, getting your own way or not getting your own way?

Client: Now there's a question. I can't really say. I've always assumed I wanted to get my own way, but I can see that if you always get your own way, you might end up being pushy like my sister.

Therapist: As opposed to . . .?

Client: (after a long silence) I suppose the issue for me is being accepted.

Therapist: Can I check back? You seem to be saying that if you don't get your own way, you are more likely to be accepted. Is the opposite also true? That if you do get your own way, you're likely to be rejected?

Client: Definitely.

Therapist: Let's look at that more specifically. Can you think of someone other than your sister who likes to get their own way?

Client: (long pause) Yes . . . a friend of mine, Nick.

Therapist: Tell me a bit about him.

Client: I know what you're getting at. (Smile) He is accepted!

Therapist: So perhaps we have to differentiate between your sister getting her own way and other people getting their own way? What was specially bad for you about your sister getting her own way?

Client: It's to do with my parents. She got her own way because she shouted the loudest and the longest. I didn't want to be that way, and I got ignored. It was difficult. (long silence)

Therapist: So you had a dilemma. You wanted things, but couldn't ask for them. Is that true of you today?

Client: I suppose so.

Therapist: Any ideas how other people get what they want and are still acceptable by and large?

This conversation makes explicit a very important construct for the client: *accepted—rejected*. Through the controlled elaboration he discovered that his assumption, that is, if you stuck out for what you wanted you would be rejected, was only true at home and probably only when he was young. The way was clear to test this and, it was hoped, reconstrue.

(ii) Problem clarification

Although other therapy models do not refer to controlled elaboration, the same sorts of strategies are used to help clients define what is bothering them. The following list of questions may be useful to therapists:

1 Tell me what you mean when you say . . .

2 Tell me about a specific instance . . .

3 How would you prefer to handle the situation?

4 What would the advantages be of . . .?

5 What will you have to do in order to . . .?

(iii) Interviewing skills with families

We have discussed the importance that we attach to developing a partnership with clients and we realise that, for some therapists, this will lead to a modification in their approach to interviewing. We would recommend experimenting with this new approach before trying it with clients. Enactment may be a useful way of exploring different styles of interviewing, since both the therapist and client roles can be experienced.

1 *The 'expert' model:* With a colleague, conduct an interview where the therapist asks a great number of questions and then, at the end, advises the parents how to behave in relation to their stuttering child. Discuss how this felt for both therapist and parent. Who had the power during the interview?

Questions for the 'mother':

■ What was it like being questioned and not knowing the purpose of the questions or how the answers would be used?

■ Did the advice make you feel optimistic about helping your child?

■ Were you able to formulate and ask questions of the therapist?

Questions for the therapist:

■ How did it feel to ask a lot of questions?

■ How easy or difficult was it to arrive at some relevant advice?

2 *The 'partnership' model:* Enact an interview where the therapist aims to establish a relationship of mutual respect. Allow the questions to develop from the content of the interview, exploring tentative hypotheses as they emerge. If possible, arrange that a few colleagues observe the interview: while watching, they can formulate hypotheses, and if the interviewer gets stuck they can all discuss how to proceed or make suggestions about which hypotheses to test with further questioning.

Interviewing a couple or family can be much more stressful than interviewing just one person. Family therapists use role-play to practise and develop these skills. Working in this way serves two important functions: first, therapists become used to being observed and second, they get experience at carrying out the suggestions that come from the observer/ supervisor. Working with families may deskill therapists, especially when they abandon the familiar structure provided by an interview questionnaire. The feelings of threat and uncertainty can be paralysing. Practice at this approach is probably the best preparation for the real event, but not necessarily the most enjoyable. It is not pleasant to appear inept in front of colleagues, but openness about the difficulties will increase therapists' skills and understanding in the long term. For those who wish to take these suggestions further, **Haley** (1976) devotes a chapter in his book to training therapists.

When interviewing families, it is useful to have some principles in mind that guide the flow of questions. The following points may be helpful:

■ Ask questions that clarify understanding.

■ Check how constructs influence behaviour. For example, if the mother talks about the child being nervous, how does she recognise that the child is nervous? What is it that the child does?

■ Observe the family actually interacting, rather than asking them how they usually interact.

■ Try to get precise examples of how parents respond to the child's problem behaviours: what do they do? What happens then?

■ In order to discover family constructs, negotiate the opposites to terms that are frequently used. Where do different members of the family place themselves along these dimensions? For example, who will be most pleased if the child stops stuttering?

(iv) Self-disclosure

We are including a few comments here on self-disclosure, because so often interviewing implies that one person questions another, and that information flows in one direction only. Occasionally it may be encouraging or supportive to disclose a personal anecdote. For example, recently a group were working on increasing their assertiveness. One client said that he felt he had such a long way to go and did not think he would ever feel assertive inside. The therapist told him how poorly she had handled things a few years back, and that experience and practice had helped her not only to be more assertive but to feel it as well. The client seemed very encouraged, and asked questions about the therapist's learning process.

This tactic needs to be handled with caution. While it certainly demonstrates empathy, it may allow the client to focus attention away from self for a while and deny the opportunity to learn. In group situations particularly, what may be good for one person may not be good for others. It is difficult to know how to judge when to use self-disclosure, but a good general rule is that if it adds something to the therapy that could not be gained otherwise, it is probably appropriate.

(c) Developing group therapy skills

The group leader has more opportunity than anyone else to influence the nature of the experience had by its membership. Thus group workers bear special responsibilities to the group and its members. In the first instance, the leader has an obligation to do everything possible to make the experience constructive and productive for each person. This implies that, during sessions, the therapist needs to note what is going on, to anticipate the consequences of her own behaviour and to modify her behaviour accordingly. Secondly, the outcome of therapy is in part the therapist's responsibility. The therapist may not be able to determine the outcome, but she certainly can influence it. Thirdly, the therapist is partly responsible for what happens during sessions. To summarise, anything that the therapist can influence is her responsibility (**Whitaker**, 1985, pp 378–9).

In order to increase the effectiveness of her approach, the group therapist needs to keep in touch with the group as a whole, with each member and with herself. The power of observation is the most important skill required in working to this end. At first the therapist may be overwhelmed by the quantity of things to observe, but in time she can try to develop a conceptual framework to structure her observations. Collecting information via careful observation is necessary if problems in the group process are to be diagnosed. Having a usable and accessible framework for understanding such problems will enable the therapist to intervene in order to change the way in which the group is working.

What should be observed? **Douglas** (1976, pp80–1) suggests the following check-list, which seems useful not only for therapists and clients, but also for structuring student speech therapists' observation of the group process:

Atmosphere	Warm, friendly, informal?
	Is there good group morale?
	Are members sensitive to the feelings of others?
Tempo	Too slow?
	Too hurried?

Continued overleaf

Interest level	High, medium, low?
	Are many people bored?
	Are there any signs of fatigue?
	Are people really interested in the topic under discussion?
Content	Is discussion specific and practical, or theoretical?
Progress	Is the problem clearly understood?
	Is there decision on possible steps to be taken in solving the problem?
	Are major points jotted down to assist the group in crystallising its thinking?
Participation	Is the discussion monopolised by a few people?
	Do some people attempt to dominate?
	Are there some persons who never say anything?
	Does any member of the group set himself up as an expert and try to answer all questions?
	Is there merely a series of speeches?
	Do persons communicate effectively?
	Are contributions brief and to the point?
	Is there an honest effort to understand each other's point of view?
	Are roles assumed by members, such as clarifier, summariser, encourager, humorist, initiator, realist, needed?

When using this type of questionnaire, it may be helpful to specify the criteria by which terms are used. For example, what made people feel that the atmosphere in the group was warm? What made people feel that the tempo was too slow? This can expand the discussion if the questionnaire is given to speech therapy students or to group members to diagnose problems in the group process. Usually such problems involve conflict, apathy or inadequate decision making (**Douglas**, 1976). Many of the situations which are seen as difficult present the therapist with an opportunity to help the group become more constructive than previously.

For example, whether or not to deal with members of the group who talk a lot can pose the therapist with an interesting dilemma. If the group is very quiet generally, it can be a great relief to the therapist if someone always initiates discussions and keeps them going. However, the other side is that as long as one person talks and takes risks, no one else has to. The sudden surge of fluency that happens to some people in stuttering groups can lead to monopolising behaviour. It is very often up to the therapist to say something like, 'I can't help noticing that Norman has been talking a lot since the start of the session. He hasn't really been sticking to the subject we were discussing. How does everyone feel about this?' When making this type of intervention, the therapist is taking a risk herself, and needs to be prepared to take the consequences of not being supported by the group. On a recent intensive course the therapist raised this issue after a role-play situation where one person had dominated the role-play and had not let the others in. David, the person thus confronted, became angry and almost tearful, saying that he would not speak again, that he had been trying to be challenging and, after all, it was up to each person to interrupt if they wanted to speak. Tom, the person who had been left out, shrugged his shoulders and said that he had not had much to say anyway. It was very difficult for the therapist to retrieve the error and re-establish her relationship with the group. 'A problem clearly lies in the eye of the beholder' (**Whitaker**, 1985, p317).

Another example of problem behaviour occurs when a person slips into the role of 'scapegoat'. Sometimes that person offers themselves up for the role, but at other times the rest of the group force the issue. In an evening class, Clive became the scapegoat. He became all things bad in the group, whose other members saw him as different. By Clive's becoming the scapegoat, the other members were able to establish close relationships with each other that excluded him. Often, when he spoke, the group gave clear signals that they were not really interested. The others did not enjoy pairing up with him when the group was split into subgroups. When we raised the issue with the group, Clive said that what was happening in the group reflected exactly what happened to him in other situations, such as at work where no one spoke to him. Clive left our therapy group, writing us a long letter ensuring our guilt by thanking the group for its support and help. On reflection, Clive was scapegoated because he refused to support the group norms, always taking an opposing stance. His refusal to conform cost him support, and members felt justified in feeling angry with him. If this had been noted early enough by the therapist a timely intervention might have changed the rather sad outcome. The nature of this intervention might have been to ask the group for instances of non-conformist behaviour on their parts and to examine its purpose and outcome. Trying to help the scapegoat to conform is counterproductive to the group process, and merely serves to maintain the role in disguised terms (**Whitaker**, 1985).

These two examples illustrate the sort of problems that may arise in groups. The vulnerability of the therapist, and the consequences of an intervention going wrong, cannot be ignored. In order to develop therapy skills and feel supported while so doing can only be achieved by having adequate supervision or at least sharing the running of the group with a co-worker. Self-awareness is an essential ingredient for growth and development as a therapist. The ability to know and be honest about feelings can facilitate the supervision process and increase the therapist's effectiveness.

Keeping in touch with her own feelings can provide the therapist with guidelines as to how the rest of the group are feeling. If the therapist is unable or unwilling to acknowledge her own feelings, these may emerge in unintended ways and hamper the group process. Before elaborating on what sorts of feelings therapists might experience in relation to groups, it is important to stress that feelings are highly subjective and do not necessarily correspond to reality. 'Feelings are not infallible' (**Johnson and Johnson**, 1982, p456). They are useful for helping the therapist to generate hypotheses which then may be tested behaviourally. Observing the outcome of her intervention on the group is a useful way of verifying the accuracy of the feelings underlying her contribution. With experience and regular self-evaluation, a therapist may learn which feelings and intuitions to trust and, conversely, when to move cautiously in relation to her inner subjective reactions.

Returning now to the nature of the feelings the therapist may experience: before the group begins, the therapist may entertain hopes for herself, which are likely to be accompanied by their polar opposites, namely, fears. There are likely to be times during the course of the group meeting when the issues the group are discussing touch on problems that the therapist is currently dealing with. At such times it may be difficult for the therapist not to exploit the group for her own ends.

There are many threats in being 'new at the game' of group therapy. A group is somehow a more public place and making mistakes is more risky than in one-to-one therapy. **Meyer Williams** (1966, quoted in **Whitaker** p217) speaks of 'fearful fantasies' among less experienced therapists: 'encountering unmanageable resistance, losing control of the group, excessive hostility breaking out, acting out by group members, overwhelming dependency demands, and group disintegration'. Most therapists worry about attendance, about getting people to speak in the group and about their own performance.

During sessions feelings of anger or confusion or even exhilaration may be aroused by the way in which the group is working. No group therapist can insulate herself against feelings. To do so would involve being distant and the possibility of losing touch with the group. The best way of dealing with powerful feelings of this sort is to decide on and maintain a helpful stance in relation to the group. The stance a therapist assumes determines the level and nature of the participation she has in the group (**Whitaker**, 1985). One test of the leader is the temptation to become 'one of the group'. However, groups need leaders to maintain the group structure and to direct the work towards its goals (**Freeman**, 1987).

The therapist is in a unique position to hold a view of the group that is mindful of how events affect each person present, because her reasons for being there are different from those of other participants. This implies that the therapist should put her own needs and concerns aside while the group is in session, and spend her time monitoring and responding to the group process. What is not implied is that the therapist holds herself remote from the group or seems cold and dispassionate. *Staying with* the group, with their feelings and issues, requires both warmth and empathy and will be noted by the group, even if the therapist says little. Many a therapist has a need to join in that probably stems from their isolation from the companionship and warmth generated in the group. Again this underlines the need for therapists to have adequate supervision, where they can offload their problems and concerns (**Freeman**, 1987).

The therapist can never lose sight of her leadership role. Group members may be late, lapse into silence or sabotage the efforts of the group, but the therapist may not do likewise. Members of the group may indicate their like or dislike of others. They may be forgiven for talking too much or too little, but not so the therapist. The group may criticise the therapist, or a number leave the group altogether. No matter how destructive a group is towards the therapist, Freeman advises, 'Never cry in the group, whatever happens—you can always cry on the way home'.

After all is said and done, leaders have an important role in groups. While they are in a powerful position to influence the interaction and achievements of the group, the group also has responsibilities of its own. Therapy can be seen as a joint venture (**Kelly**, 1955) and this implies sharing the successes and failures of the group. Freeman points out how quick groups are to congratulate themselves if all goes well, and how quickly they blame the leader if it does not!

Is there such a thing as an ideal group therapist? Not really. Different groups call for different qualities at different times. The capacity of therapists to vary their style in relation to the needs of a group is likely to be a determining factor of their success as group leaders. Careful and critical appraisal of their efforts on their own and with their supervisors, transforms mere experience into constructive learning and personal growth and development.

(d) Tasks for group therapists

(i) Planning and designing a course of therapy

As an exercise, it may be useful to plan a course of group therapy for each of the following:

- Establishment of fluency for adults
- Two-week intensive course for 13–16 year olds
- Maintenance of change for adults who have had block modification therapy.

The headings given below may be helpful:

- Aims and objectives of the course,
- Selection criteria and numbers,
- Frequency and length of sessions,
- Setting,
- Duration of the course,
- Leadership: single or joint,
- Activities to be used,
- Special techniques to be used,
- Evaluation of effectiveness of the course,
- Arrangements for supervision.

(ii) What sort of leader am I?

This question could equally be rephrased as 'What sort of leader would I like to be?' Connecting the style of leadership to the aims of the group is an important part of the planning process. The questions below may serve to structure self-appraisal:

- What powers do I or don't I have?
- What responsibilities do I or don't I have?
- What sort of leadership role would be most useful to this group?

- What are my strengths as a group therapist?
- What aspects of my behaviour do I have to monitor or modify?
- How will I know if I'm doing a good job?
- What support do I need?

(iii) Dealing with problems in the group

Every group has its problems. Being prepared for potential problems may lead to a more satisfactory solution than if the therapist is taken by surprise. Use the list of common group problems that follows as the basis for deciding what stance to take if they occur.

- Conflicts of interest where one person blocks or makes the actions of another person less effective.
- Lack of co-operation from the group.
- Violation of the group rules or norms.
- Over-talkative members.
- Refusal to participate in an exercise.
- Attack on the therapist.
- A persistently silent person.
- Sexist or racist remarks.
- Frequent absences.
- Scapegoating.
- Stereotyping of one member into role of clown, for example.
- A sexual relationship developing between two members.
- Changing membership.
- Where the aims no longer serve the needs of the group members.

(iv) Dependency and counter-dependency

In any form of therapy it is likely that the client becomes dependent on the therapist and that the therapist in turn uses the relationship to meet some of her own needs. Dependency has to be dealt with if the aims of therapy are to be realised, that is, that the client may leave therapy having changed and is able to have his dependency needs met outside. As part of the process of evaluating therapy and the therapist's role, answering the following questions may give the therapist direction in dealing with the very human issue of dependency.

- How do I relate to each member of the group?
- Are my actions always in the interests of promoting change in the client?
- Am I flattered by anyone's opinion of me?
- Do I seek approval from anyone in the group?
- How do I feel about the group coming to an end?
- Do I wish to change my relationship with anyone in the group to friendship?
- Are my needs being met outside the group?

Although the answers to such questions are not always pleasant, it is necessary to ask them.

Supervision

Throughout this book we have urged therapists to seek supervision for themselves, not as a luxury, but as a necessary part of their personal growth and development. We see supervision as a learning relationship: therapists set aside time to discover more about their personal strengths and weaknesses, and also to find ways of overcoming problems. It probably goes without saying that supervision will be most helpful if the supervisor has experience and skills both as a therapist and as a supervisor. In our profession this is not always possible, and we may like to turn to social workers or psychologists for help initially. If possible, the person chosen to supervise should not be able to use their position to influence or manipulate the other.

We strongly recommend that supervision be regarded as part and parcel of a therapist's normal working hours. The frequency and length of sessions will depend on what arrangements can be made in each individual case. The recommended frequency and length are weekly sessions that last 45–60 minutes (**Munro, Manthei and Small**, 1983).

The content of supervision must be negotiated between the therapist and her supervisor. We recommend that not all the time is spent diagnosing the client's problems, but rather the discussion should focus on the therapist's ways of helping the client: the personal threats and areas of anxiety. The emphasis needs to be on the personal aspects of therapy, otherwise the only benefit from supervision will be that the therapist gets better at diagnosing other people's problems. A further focus in sessions should be on the skills involved in the therapy process. For example, if a therapist is wary about confronting a particular client, she may like to role play the situation during supervision. During supervision, therapists are likely to be encouraged to evaluate themselves, to say what they feel about themselves as therapists. In this sense, supervision is not unlike having therapy, and can provide the therapist with insight and understanding of the process of change. Sessions are likely to end with some aims and objectives for the therapist to pursue, again much like a therapy session.

Sometimes therapists may attend a supervision group, where they each take turns to present problems or raise issues that have generality to the group. For therapists who are comfortable in groups, and who are able to take risks, this can be very advantageous. For others it might increase their sense of vulnerability. There is no ideal; each therapist must choose for themselves.

If it is not possible to arrange supervision, what are the alternatives? Within the speech therapy profession there is potential for a support structure that may be helpful. Less experienced therapists may turn to their seniors for advice and help with certain problems. This cannot be seen as a substitute for formal supervision, but at least it enables therapists to ask questions and to evaluate their work.

Mutual supervision can be arranged where a group of colleagues contract with each other to meet on a regular basis and discuss therapy issues. Ground rules are necessary to maximise use of time. We have been running a mutual supervision group over the last five years. There have been problems and distractions, but creating time to talk about therapy matters with each other has been constructive. The ground rules that we try to adhere to are as follows:

- We will meet once a week for an hour.
- The time will not be used for moaning.
- Nor will it be used to gossip, socialise or discuss other matters.
- In the supervision group we will work on a non-hierarchical basis.
- Everyone will be given equal time to discuss issues.

- We will endeavour to listen constructively.
- There is no obligation to carry out suggestions made.

Other than these ground rules, sessions are similar to those described at the start of the section on supervision. Mutual supervision should be encouraging and afford therapists an opportunity to evaluate their work and identify areas to change.

Conclusion

As we indicated in our introduction, writing this book has taken us on a journey through our confusions about stuttering. Trying to elaborate why we do what we do has helped us to clarify our thoughts about stuttering and what we believe constitutes satisfactory therapy. However, knowing how we view the problem and why we choose particular ways of approaching it, has placed us on the edge of a new horizon: answers beget more questions, and so the process begins again . . .

GLOSSARY OF TERMS*

Formal aspects of constructs

Contrast. The relationship between the two poles of a construct is one of contrast.

Elements. The things or events which are abstracted by a person's use of a construct are called elements. In some systems these are called objects.

Emergence. The emergent pole of a construct is that one which embraces most of the immediately perceived context.

Implicitness. The implicit pole of a construct is that one which embraces contrasting context. It contrasts with the emergent pole. Frequently the person has no available symbol or name for it; it is symbolised only implicitly by the emergent term.

Permeability. A construct is permeable if it admits newly perceived elements to its context. It is impermeable if it rejects elements on the basis of their newness.

Pole. Each construct discriminates between two poles, one at each end of its dichotomy. The elements abstracted are like each other at each pole with respect to the construct and are unlike the elements at the other pole.

Range of convenience. A construct's range of convenience comprises all those things to which the user would find its application useful.

Constructs classified according to the nature of their control over their elements

Constellatory construct. A construct which fixes the other realm memberships of its elements is called a constellatory construct. This is stereotyped or typological thinking.

Pre-emptive construct. A construct which pre-empts its elements for membership in its own realm exclusively is called a pre-emptive construct. This is the 'nothing but' type of construction – 'If this is a ball it is nothing but a ball.'

Propositional construct. A construct which carries no implications regarding the other realm memberships of its elements is a propositional construct. This is uncontaminated construction.

General diagnostic constructs

Comprehensive constructs. A comprehensive construct is one which subsumes a wide variety of events.

Constriction. Constriction occurs when a person narrows his perceptual field in order to minimise apparent incompatibilities.

Core constructs. A core construct is one which governs the client's maintenance processes.

---

* *All of these definitions are derived directly or indirectly from Kelly (1955)*

Dilation. Dilation occurs when a person broadens his perceptual field in order to reorganise it on a more comprehensive level. It does not, in itself, include the comprehensive reconstruction of those elements.

Incidental constructs. An incidental construct is one which subsumes a narrow variety of events.

Level of cognitive awareness. The level of cognitive awareness ranges from high to low. A high-level construct is one which is readily expressed in socially effective symbols; whose alternatives are both readily accessible; which falls well within the range of convenience of the client's major constructions; and which is not suspended by its superordinating constructs.

Loose constructs. A loose construct is one leading to varying predictions, but which retains its identity.

Peripheral constructs. A peripheral construct is one which can be altered without serious modification of the core structure.

Preverbal constructs. A preverbal construct is one which continues to be used, even though it has no consistent word symbol. It may or may not have been devised before the client had command of speech symbolism.

Submergence. The submerged pole of a construct is the one which is less available for application to events.

Subordinate constructs. A subordinate construct is one which is included as an element in the context of another.

Superordinate constructs. A superordinate construct is one which includes another as one of the elements in its context.

Suspension. A suspended element is one which is omitted from the context of a construct as a result of revision of the client's construct system.

Tight constructs. A tight construct is one which leads to unvarying predictions.

Constructs relating to transition

Aggressiveness. Aggressiveness is the active elaboration of one's perceptual field.

Anxiety. Anxiety is the awareness that the events with which one is confronted lie mostly outside the range of convenience of his construct system.

C-P-C cycle. The C-P-C cycle is a sequence of construction involving, in succession, circumspection, pre-emption and control, and leading to a choice precipitating the person into a particular situation.

Fear. Fear is the awareness of an imminent incidental change in one's core structures.

Guilt. Guilt is the awareness of dislodgement of the self from one's core role structure.

Hostility. Hostility is the continued effort to extort validational evidence in favour of a type of social prediction which has already been recognised as a failure.

Impulsivity. Impulsivity is a characteristic foreshortening of the C-P-C cycle.

Threat. Threat is the awareness of imminent comprehensive change in one's core structures.

Other terms used

Constructive alternativism. We assume that all of our present interpretations of the universe are subject to revision or replacement.

Construing. Construing means placing an interpretation upon events in order to make sense of them. To this end, we evolve a structure (that is, a construct system) within which the events we encounter make sense. The process of construing involves noting similarities and differences in any series of events. Construing is not the same as verbal formulation, and may occur at different levels of cognitive awareness.

Events. Kelly's use of the term 'events' is somewhat esoteric. He does not refer just to 'happenings', but to anything that can be construed. This includes people, the things people do, situations, time, and so on.

Invalidation. Invalidation represents incompatibility between one's prediction and the observed outcome.

Prediction. Constructs form the basis of predictions. When we make a prediction, we anticipate some of the properties of the event, rather than every last detail. For example, the experience of learning in school enables us to make predictions about the nature of higher education. The constructs we have evolved in the school situation will be useful to us in choosing how to behave when we come to make the transition from school to university.

Validation. Validation refers solely to the verification of a prediction. In this way it differs from the concept of 'reinforcement' because predictions of both good and bad events can be validated.

BIBLIOGRAPHY

Andrews G and **Cutler J**, 'Stuttering Therapy: the Relation between Changes in Symptom Level and Attitudes', *Journal of Speech and Hearing Disorders*, 39, pp312–19, 1974.

Bannister D, 'A New Theory of Personality', Foss B M (ed), *New Horizons in Psychology* 1, Penguin Books, Harmondsworth, 1966.

Bannister D and **Agnew J**, 'The Child's Construing of Self', Landfield A W (ed), *1976 Nebraska Symposium on Motivation*, University of Nebraska Press, Lincoln, 1977.

Bannister D and **Fransella F**, *Inquiring Man*, Croom Helm, London, 1986.

Bannister D and **Higginbotham P G**, *The GAB Computer Program for the Analysis of Repertory Grid Data*, Second Edition, 1983.

Barker P, *Basic Family Therapy*, Collins, London, 1986.

Beck A, Ward C, Mendelsohn M, Mock J and **Erbaugh J**, 'An Inventory for Measuring Depression', *Archives of General Psychiatry*, 4, pp561–71, 1961.

Beveridge M and **Brierley C**, 'Classroom Constructs: An Interpretive Approach to Young Children's Language', Beveridge M, (ed), *Children Thinking Through Language*, Edward Arnold, London, 1982.

Blood G W and **Seider R**, 'The Concommitant Problems of Young Stutterers', *Journal of Speech and Hearing Disorders* 46, pp31–3, 1981.

Bloodstein O and **Grossman M**, 'Early Stutterings: Some Aspects of Their Form and Distribution', *Journal of Speech and Hearing Research* 24, pp298–302, 1981.

Boberg E, *Maintenance of Fluency: Proceedings of the Banff Conference*, Elsevier, Amsterdam, 1981.

Boberg E and **Kully D**, *Comprehensive Stuttering Program: Clinical Manual*, Taylor and Francis, New York, 1985.

Brammer L M and **Shostrom E L**, *Therapeutic Psychology*, Prentice-Hall, New Jersey, 1968.

Brandes D and **Phillips H**, *Gamesters' Handbook*, Hutchinson, London, 1978.

Broverman I K, Broverman D M, Clarkson F E, Rosenkrantz P and **Vogel S R**, 'Sex Role Stereotypes and Clinical Judgements of Mental Health', *Journal of Consulting Psychology* 34, pp1–7, 1970.

Brutten G, 'Stuttering: Topography, Assessment and Behaviour Change Strategies', Eisenson J (ed), *Stuttering: A Second Symposium*, Harper and Row, New York, 1975.

Byrne R, 'Individual Therapy with the Very Severe Stutterer', Levy C (ed), *Stuttering Therapies: Practical Approaches*, Croom Helm, London, 1987.

Cheasman C, 'Therapy for Adults: an Evaluation of Current Techniques for Establishing Fluency', Dalton P (ed), *Approaches to the Treatment of Stuttering*, Croom Helm, London, 1983.

Cheasman C, 'Personal Communication', paper presented at City Lit, 1986.

Cheasman C, 'An Overview of Issues in Therapy with Adults who Stutter', Levy C (ed), *Stuttering Therapies: Practical Approaches*, Croom Helm, London, 1987.

Clezy G, *Modification of the Mother–Child Interchange in Language, Speech and Hearing,* Edward Arnold, London, 1979.

Clifford J and **Watson P,** 'Family Counselling with Children who Stutter: an Adlerian Approach', Levy C (ed), *Stuttering Therapies: Practical Approaches,* Croom Helm, London, 1987.

Cooper E and **Cooper C,** *Cooper Personalised Fluency Control Therapy—Revised,* DLM Teaching Resources, Texas, 1985.

Costello J, 'Current Behavioural Treatments for Children', Prins D and Ingham R (eds), *Treatment of Stuttering in Early Childhood: Methods and Issues,* College-Hill Press, California, 1983.

Cox G and **Dainow S,** *Making the Most of Yourself,* Sheldon Press, London, 1985.

Crowe B, *Play is a Feeling,* Unwin Paperbacks, London, 1983.

Cunningham C and **Davis H,** *Working with Parents: Frameworks for Collaboration,* Open University Press, 1985.

Dalton P, 'A Personal Construct Therapy Approach to Therapy with Children', Edwards G (ed), *Current Issues in Clinical Psychology,* Plenum Publications, New York, 1986.

Dalton P, 'Some Developments in Personal Construct Therapy with Adults who Stutter', Levy C (ed), *Stuttering Therapies: Practical Approaches,* Croom Helm, London, 1987a.

Dalton P, 'One Way of Construing Relationships', *Constructs,* vol. 5, no. 3, p 3, 1987b.

Dare C, 'Psychoanalysis and Systems in Family Therapy', *Journal of Family Therapy,* 1, pp137–51, 1979.

De Joy D and **Gregory H,** 'The Relationship between Age and Frequency of Disfluency in Preschool Children', *Journal of Fluency Disorders* 10, pp107–22, 1985.

Douglas T, *Groupwork Practice,* Tavistock Publications, London, 1976.

Douglas T, *Basic Groupwork,* Tavistock Publications, London, 1978.

Egolf D, Shames G, Johnson P and **Kasprisin-Burrelli A,** 'The Use of Parent–Child Interaction in Therapy for Young Stutterers', *Journal of Speech and Hearing Disorders* 37, 2, pp222–32, 1972.

Epting F, *Personal Construct Counselling and Psychotherapy,* John Wiley and Sons, New York, 1984.

Epting F and **Amerikaner M,** 'Optimal Functioning: A Personal Construct Approach', Landfield, A W and Leitner L M (eds) *Personal Construct Psychology: Psychotherapy and Personality,* John Wiley and Sons, New York, 1980.

Evesham M, 'Residential Courses for Stutterers: Combining Technique and Personal Construct Psychology', Levy C (ed), *Stuttering Therapies: Practical Approaches,* Croom Helm, London, 1987.

Evesham M and **Fransella F,** 'Stuttering Relapse: the Effect of Combined Speech and Psychological Reconstruction Programme', *British Journal of Disorders of Communication* 20, pp237–48, 1985.

Fransella F, 'Self Constructs and the Stutterer', *British Journal of Psychiatry* 114, pp1531–5, 1968.

Fransella F, 'Stuttering: Not a Symptom but a Way of Life', *British Journal of Disorders of Communication* 5, pp22–9, 1970.

Fransella F, *Personal Change and Reconstruction,* Academic Press, London, 1972.

Fransella F, 'Personal Construct Therapy', Dryden W (ed), *Individual Therapy in Britain,* Harper and Row, New York, 1984.

Fransella F and **Bannister D,** *A Manual for Repertory Grid Technique,* Academic Press, London, 1977.

Fraser J, *Stuttering Therapy: Transfer and Maintenance,* Speech Foundation of America, Memphis, Tennessee, 1984.

Freeman R, 'Leadership in Small Groups', *Horizons* 1, 6, pp299–304, 1987.

Goldman-Eisler F, *Psycholinguistics: Experiments in Spontaneous Speech,* Academic Press, London, 1968.

Gordon P, Luper H and **Peterson H,** 'The Effects of Syntactic Complexity on the Occurrence of Disfluencies in Five Year Old Non-stutterers', *Journal of Fluency Disorders* 11, pp151–64, 1986.

Gregory H H, *Controversies About Stuttering Therapy,* University Park Press, Baltimore, 1979.

Gregory H H, 'Prevention of Stuttering: Management of Early Stages', Curlee R F and Perkins W H (eds), *Nature and Treatment of Stuttering: New Directions,* Taylor and Francis, New York, 1985.

Gregory H H, 'Environmental Manipulation and Family Counselling', Shames G H and Rubin H (eds), *Stuttering Then and Now,* Charles E Merrill Publishing Company, Columbus, Ohio, 1986.

Haley J, *Problem-Solving Therapy,* Harper Torch Books, New York, 1976.

Hayhow R, 'The Assessment of Stuttering and the Evaluation of Treatment', Dalton P (ed), *Approaches to the Treatment of Stuttering,* Croom Helm, London, 1983.

Hayhow R, 'Personal Construct Theory and Motherhood', unpublished diploma thesis, Centre for Personal Construct Psychology, 1986.

Hayhow R, 'Personal Construct Therapy with Children who Stutter and Their Families', Levy C (ed), *Stuttering Therapies: Practical Approaches,* Croom Helm, London, 1987.

Heinze B and **Johnson K,** *Easy Does It,* Lingui Systems, Illinois, 1985.

Helps R and **Dalton P,** 'The Effectiveness of an Intensive Group Therapy Programme for Adult Stammerers', *British Journal of Disorders of Communication* 14, 17–30, 1979.

Hinkle D, 'The Change of Personal Constructs from the Viewpoint of a Theory of Construct Implications', unpublished PhD thesis, Ohio State University, 1965.

Hughes S, *Dogger,* Collins Picture Lions, London, 1979.

Hughes S, *Moving Molly,* Collins Picture Lions, London, 1981.

Hughes S, *Alfie's Feet,* Collins Picture Lions, London, 1984.

Jackson S, 'Self Characterisation: Dimensions and Meaning', *Paper Presented at the Sixth International Congress of Personal Construct Psychology,* Cambridge, England, 1985.

Jackson S and **Bannister D,** 'Growing into Self', Bannister D (ed), *Issues and Approaches in Personal Construct Theory,* Academic Press, London, 1985a.

Jackson S and **Bannister D,** 'The Development of Self Construing in Children', unpublished paper, 1985b.

Johnson D W and **Johnson F P,** *Joining Together: Group Theory and Group Skills,* Prentice-Hall, Englewood Cliffs, NJ, 1975 and 1982.

Johnson W *et al.,* *The Onset of Stuttering,* Minneapolis University Press, Minnesota, 1959.

Kelly G A, *The Psychology of Personal Constructs,* Norton Press, New York, 1955.

Kelly G A, 'Ontological Acceleration', Maher B (ed), *Clinical Psychology and Personality,* Robert E Krieger Publishing Company, New York, 1969.

Kelly G A, 'Behaviour is an Experiment', Bannister D (ed), *Perspectives in Personal Construct Theory,* Academic Press, London, 1970.

Kelly G A, 'A Psychology of Optimal Man', Landfield A W and Leitner, L M (eds), *Personal Construct Psychology: Psychotherapy and Personality,*

John Wiley and Sons, New York, 1980.

Laing R D, *Knots,* Penguin Books, Harmondsworth, 1972.

Landfield A W, *Personal Construct Systems in Psychotherapy,* McNally Rand, New York, 1971.

Landfield A W and **Epting F,** *Personal Construct Psychology: Clinical and Personality Assessment,* Human Sciences Press, New York, 1987.

Leitner L M, 'Psychopathology and the differentiation of values, emotions and behaviours: a repertory grid study, *British Journal of Psychiatry* 138, pp147–53, 1981.

Leitner L M, 'Interview Methodologies for Construct Elicitation: Searching for the Core', Epting F and Landfield A W, (eds), *Anticipating Personal Construct Psychology,* University of Nebraska Press, Lincoln, 1985.

Levy C, 'Interiorised Stuttering: A Group Therapy Approach', Levy C (ed), *Stuttering Therapies: Practical Approaches,* Croom Helm, London, 1987.

Levy C and **Insley T,** 'The demands—and rewards—of co-therapy', *Speech Therapy in Practice* vol. 3, no. 1, p 7, 1987.

Mareck J and **Johnson M,** 'Gender and the Process of Therapy', *Women and Psychotherapy,* The Guildford Press, New York, 1980.

Morris C, 'The use of repertory grid technique with a seven-year-old girl who has athetoid quadreplegia and severe communication disability', unpublished BSc thesis, Central School of Speech and Drama, London, 1987.

Munro E, Manthei R J and **Small J J,** *Counselling: A Skills Approach,* Methuen, New Zealand, 1983.

Murphy A and **Fitzsimmons R,** *Stuttering and Personality Dynamics,* Ronald Press, New York, 1960.

Perkins W H, 'From Psychoanalysis to Discoordination', Gregory H H (ed), *Controversies about Stuttering Therapy,* University Park Press, Baltimore, 1979.

Perkins W H, 'Onset of Stuttering: The Case of the Missing Block', Prins D and Ingham R J (eds), *The Treatment of Stuttering in Early Childhood: Methods and Issues,* College-Hill Press, California, 1983.

Pinney R, *Creative Listening,* Children's Hour Trust, 1983.

Pinney R, Carr-Gomm P and **Robinson M,** *Special Times—Listening to Children,* Children's Hour Trust, 1985.

Pollack J, Lubinsky R and **Weitzner-Lin B,** 'A Pragmatic Study of Child Disfluency', *Journal of Fluency Disorders* 11, pp231–9, 1986.

Price H, 'Depression, Anxiety and Locus of Control in Adults who Stutter', unpublished BSc thesis, Central School of Speech and Drama, London, 1987.

Prins D, 'Continuity, Fragmentation and Tension', Prins D and Ingham R J (eds), *Treatment of Stuttering in Early Childhood: Methods and Issues,* College-Hill Press, California, 1983.

Procter H, 'A Construct Approach to Family Therapy and Systems Intervention', Button E (ed), *Personal Construct Theory and Mental Health,* Croom Helm, London, 1985a.

Procter H, 'The Investigation', unpublished information for students, 1985b.

Procter H, 'Change in the Family Construct System: The Therapy of a Mute and Withdrawn Schizophrenic Patient, Niemeyer R and Niemeyer G (eds), *Casebook in Personal Construct Therapy,* Springer Publishing Co., New York, 1986.

Procter H and **Walker G,** 'Brief Therapy', Street E (ed), *Family Therapy in Britain,* Harper and Row, New York, 1987.

Ravenette A T, 'Personal Construct Theory: an Approach to the Psychological Investigation of Children and Young People', Bannister D (ed), *New Perspectives in Personal Construct Theory*, Academic Press, London, 1977a.

Ravenette A T, 'Self Description Grids for Children', paper given at the Second International Congress of Personal Construct Theory, 1977b.

Ravenette A T, 'The Exploration of Consciousness: Personal Construct Intervention with Children', Landfield A W and Leitner L M (eds), *Personal Construct Psychology: Psychotherapy and Personality*, John Wiley and Sons, New York, 1980.

Ravenette A T, 'To Tell a Story, To Invent a Character, To Make a Difference', unpublished paper, London Borough of Newham.

Ravenette A T, 'Personal Construct Psychology in the Practice of an Educational Psychologist', Dunnett G (ed), *Working with People: Clinical Uses of Personal Construct Psychology*, Routledge & Kegan Paul, in press.

Reid T, 'Intensive Block Modification Therapy', Levy C (ed), *Stuttering Therapies: Practical Approaches*, Croom Helm, London, 1987.

Riley G and **Riley J,** 'A Component Model for Diagnosing and Treating Children who Stutter', *Journal of Fluency Disorders* 4, pp279–93, 1979.

Riley G and **Riley J,** 'Evaluation as a Basis for Intervention', Prins D and Ingham R J (eds), *Treatment of Stuttering in Early Childhood: Methods and Issues*, College Hill Press, California, 1983.

Rotter J, 'Generalised Expectancies for Internal vs External Control of Reinforcement', *Psychological Monograph* 80, pp1–28, 1966.

Rowe D, *Depression: The Way out of Your Prison,* Routledge & Kegan Paul, 1983.

Rustin L and **Cook F,** 'Intervention Procedures for the Disfluent Child', Dalton P (ed), *Approaches to the Treatment of Stuttering,* Croom Helm, London, 1983.

Ryan B P and **Van Kirk B,** *Monterey Fluency Program*, Monterey Learning Systems, Palo Alto, California, 1978.

St Louis K O, *The Atypical Stutterer*, Academic Press, London, 1986.

Salmon P, 'A Psychology of Personal Growth', Bannister D (ed), *Perspectives in Personal Construct Theory*, Academic Press, London, 1970.

Salmon P, 'Relations with the Physical: an Alternative Reading of Kelly', Bannister D (ed), *Issues and Approaches in Personal Construct Theory*, Academic Press, London, 1985a.

Salmon P, *Living in Time,* J M Dent, London, 1985b.

Shames G and **Florance C,** *Stutter-Free Speech: A Goal for Therapy*, Charles E Merrill Publishing Co, Columbus, 1980.

Sheehan J G, 'Conflict Theory of Stuttering', Eisenson J (ed), *Stuttering: A Symposium*, Harper and Row, New York, 1958.

Sheehan J G, 'Conflict Theory and Avoidance-Reduction Therapy', Eisenson J (ed), *Stuttering: A Second Symposium*, Harper and Row, New York, 1975.

Sheehan J G, 'Current Issues on Stuttering and Recovery', Gregory H H (ed), *Controversies about Stuttering Therapy,* University Park Press, Baltimore, 1979.

Sheehan J G, 'Theory and Treatment of Stuttering as an Approach-Avoidance Conflict', Shames G H and Rubin H (eds), *Stuttering Then and Now,* Charles E Merrill Publishing Company, Ohio, 1986.

Sheehan J G and **Sheehan V M,** 'Avoidance-Reduction Therapy: A Response-Suppression Hypothesis', Perkins W H (ed), *Stuttering Disorders*, Thieme-Stratton, New York, 1984.

Shewell M, 'The Use of Repertory Grid Technique with Children who have

Downs Syndrome', unpublished BSc thesis, Central School of Speech and Drama, London, 1987.

Shine R E, 'Direct Management of the Beginning Stutterer', *Seminars in Speech, Language and Hearing* I, pp 339–50, 1980.

Silverman E–M, 'Speech-Language Clinicians' and University Students' Impressions of Women and Girls who Stutter', *Journal of Fluency Disorders* 7, pp469–78, 1982.

Silverman E–M, 'The Female Stutterer', St Louis K O (ed), *The Atypical Stutterer*, Academic Press, London, 1986.

Silverman E–M and **Zimmer C,** 'Demographic Characteristics and Treatment Experiences of Women and Men who Stutter', *Journal of Fluency Disorders* 7, pp273–85, 1982.

Stewart T, 'Positive Attitude to Fluency: A Group Therapy Programme', Levy C (ed), *Stuttering Therapies: Practical Approaches*, Croom Helm, London, 1987a.

Stewart T, 'Personal Communication', unpublished paper, 1987b.

Stocker B and **Gerstman L,** 'A comparison of the probe technique and conventional therapy for young stutterers', *Journal of Fluency Disorders,* pp331–9, 1983.

Stournaras E F, 'A Cross-Sectional Study of Disfluencies in Speech of Normal Children aged between 2.5 and 6.2 years', paper presented at the XIX Congress of the International Association of Logopedics and Phoniatrics, 1983.

Tschudi F, 'Loaded and Honest Questions', Bannister D (ed), *New Perspectives in Personal Construct Theory,* Academic Press, London, 1977.

Turnbaugh K R, Guitar B E and **Hoffman P R,** 'The attribution of personality traits: the stutterer and the nonstutterer', *Journal of Speech and Hearing Research* 24, pp288–91, 1979.

Van Riper C, *The Treatment of Stuttering,* Prentice-Hall, Englewood Cliffs, NJ, 1973.

Wall M J and **Meyers F L,** *Clinical Management of Childhood Stuttering,* University Park Press, Baltimore, 1984.

Watzlawick P, Beavin J and **Jackson D,** *Pragmatics of Human Communication: The Study of Interactional Patterns, Pathologies and Paradoxes,* Norton, New York, 1967.

Watzlawick P, Weakland J and **Fisch R,** *Change: Principles of Problem Formation and Problem Resolution,* Norton, New York, 1974.

Wexler K and **Mysack E,** 'Disfluency Characteristics of 2-, 4-, and 6-yr-old Males', *Journal of Fluency Disorders* 7, pp37–46, 1982.

Whitaker D S, *Using Groups to Help People,* Routledge & Kegan Paul, London, 1985.

Williams D E, 'Stuttering Therapy for Children', Travis L E (ed), *Handbook of Speech Pathology*, Appleton-Century-Crofts, New York, 1971.

Williams D E, 'A Perspective on Approaches to Stuttering Therapy', Gregory H H (ed), *Controversies About Stuttering Therapy*, University Park Press, Baltimore, 1979.

Williams M, 'Limitations, fantasies, and security operations of beginning group psychotherapists', *International Journal of Group Psychotherapy* 16, pp150–62, 1966.

Yairi E, 'Disfluencies of Normally Speaking Two year old children', *Journal of Speech and Hearing Research* 24, pp490–95, 1981.